I need to look great for all patrons,

so please keep me away from food,

drinks, pets, ink, pencils, and other

things that may harm me.

"WHATEVER." JASPER JERVIS (SON)

"IT'S OK I GUESS. HE'S MY DAD." ROMY JERVIS (DAUGHTER)

"I HAD NO IDEA HE WOULD REMEMBER ANY OF THIS STUFF. I DIDN'T." JOHN JERVIS (DAD)

"I DON'T HAVE KIDS, BUT IF I DID, I'D TOTALLY TRY THIS STUFF!" WANNABE PARENT

"SO FUN! MY KIDS LOVE MATCHING SOCKS NOW. THANK YOU!" ACTUAL PARENT

"I'M JUST GLAD WE DID'NT SCREW YOU AND YOUR BROTHER UP TOO BADLY HONEY" JAN JERVIS (MOM)

Skyhorse Publishing books may be purchased in bulk at special discounts for sales promotion, corporate gifts, fund-raising, or educational purposes. Special editions can also be created to specifications. For details, contact the Special Sales Department, Skyhorse Publishing, 307 West 36th Street, 11th Floor, New York, NY 10018 or info@skyhorsepublishing.com.

Skyhorse® and Skyhorse Publishing® are registered trademarks of Skyhorse Publishing, Inc.®, a Delaware corporation.

Visit our website at www.skyhorsepublishing.com.

10 9 8 7 6 5 4 3 2 1

Library of Congress Cataloging-in-Publication Data is available on file.

Cover design by Matthew Jervis
Cover and interior illustrations by Matthew Jervis

Print ISBN: 978-1-63220-625-1
Ebook ISBN: 978-1-63220-749-4

Printed in China

How to Entertain, Distract, and Unplug Your Kids!

Tricks, Tools, and Spontaneous Screen-Free Activities

By Matthew Jervis

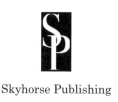

Skyhorse Publishing

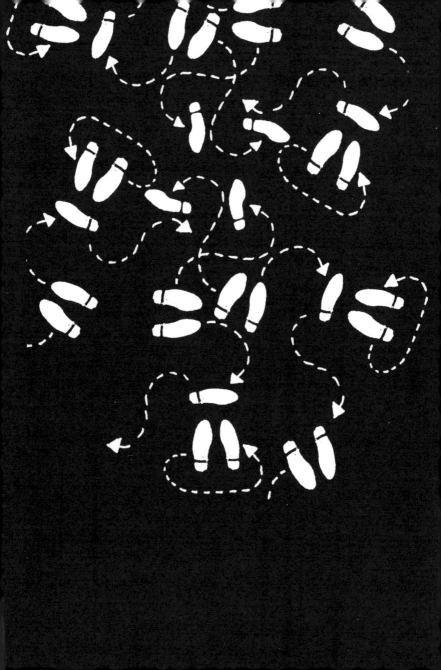

DON'T PANIC BE CREATIVE

To Romy and Jasper,
The two reasons I make anything.

TABLE OF CONTENTS

just Long Enough.

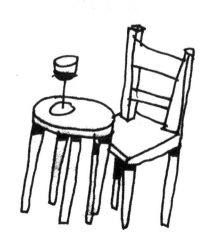

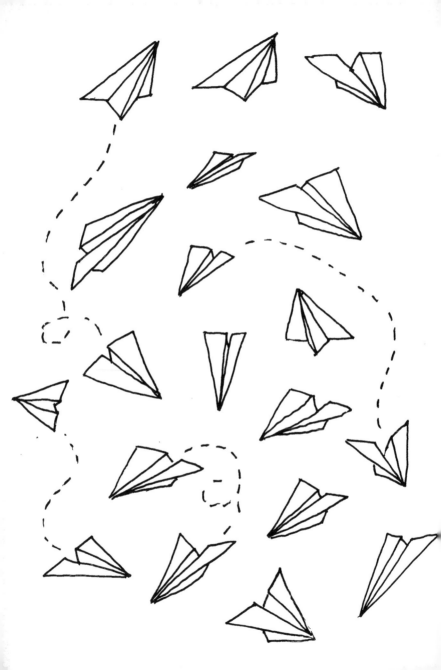

Hey there, I'm Matthew.

I'm a dad, teacher, artist, maker, and designer. So, as you can well imagine, I'm pretty busy.

I wrote this book because I love my kids and want to spend every waking minute with them, but the reality is, I can't. Sometimes Dad has to work, pay the bills, run errands, or even talk to other adults.

But still, I didn't want to just leave my kids up to their own devices . . . or mine. So I started inventing little games and projects to occupy them for twenty minutes here, an hour there.

To be truthful, my first attempts at these games were mildly wicked, like "Go find Daddy a $4 bill." Although I do offer a new take on this family favorite here in this book.

But soon, they were onto me, so I had to move beyond "impossible" tasks. And as it turns out, kids are a lot more receptive to an engaging activity than a boring boondoggle.

These days, I delight in coming up with projects to entertain, educate, and inspire kids. My own kids, and other people's.

And so I give you: *How To Entertain, Distract, and Unplug Your Kids!*

Sorry, hammer. This book will be the new favorite tool.

Enjoy.

Love,

Matthew Jervis

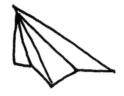

INTRODUCTION

"Dad, I'm so boooooored!"

We've all been there. Our internal record is stuck, we wander around aimlessly until we've had enough of it and knock the side of our jukebox to stop the incessant skip, and finally we find a groove and we're off and running.

Being able to whack ourselves out of boredom is a learned skill, and one that I would characterize as a pretty important one. The ability to pick ourselves up and switch our focus and move forward could be considered a survival skill!

As kids, boredom can feel like an endless slog, but with the right kind of support, they can learn to change their course on their own and not wallow in their boredom for too long.

Of course there are different kinds of boredom. First, you have that deep-seated "general apathy" kind that might require some professional help.

Then there's the kind your kid gets on a rainy afternoon. If you can get your kids to see their way through that kind, you could actually be teaching them a very important life lesson.

Self-reliance, as defined by Merriam-Webster, is "reliance on one's own efforts and abilities." When you look at it like that, being bored could be a very important teaching moment! One that requires patience and determination. We so easily give in to our kids at those moments and hand them our phone or switch on the TV, just so they stop complaining about being bored! Ugh! Who wants to hear that all day?

What we should be doing is nothing, or as little as possible; don't give in to the whining, just toss them a book and tell them, "Read your way out of it!" Or my favorite, "Only boring people get bored!"

Eventually we want them to be able to look at things a little differently so we can knock their own skipping record back into the groove. That's what I'd like this book to do. Simply help you to look at life's moments a little differently, possibly opening yourself up to seeing new opportunities so you can recognize the teaching moments that happen all the time. Raising kids is not easy, but that doesn't mean it can't be fun!

Stuck inside for the weekend? On a long car trip? Want the kids to help out? All seem just a little easier when you can see the situation as a potential adventure full of fun lessons and goofy little games that might actually teach them to be more self-reliant and creative problem solvers, when really you just want to occupy them for a couple minutes and get off your back asking to see your phone!

HISTORICALLY SPEAKING

Throughout history, parents and care-giving adults have been tasked with passing certain valuable life skills and knowledge down to the next generation. Practical skills like hunting, sharpening sticks, building fires, and folding laundry, along with more social skills like how to shake hands, make friends, and mingle at parties. Long ago these were deemed important bits of knowledge that every child would need to know in order to ensure their survival in the world.

Today, on top of all that, we're also expected to entertain our kids. We hope, mostly in vain, for some form of magic to fill in the boring bits but alas, most times it's on us to supply the "magic." What if you could combine teaching important life skills with entertainment? Maybe that sounds too lofty an idea . . . or is it?

JUST LONG ENOUGH

My brother Shawn and I were lucky enough to have spent our formative years in Colorful Colorado with two creative parents. Thing is, being a kid in that part of the country meant, in most cases, that you were at some level participating in one or more of the natural offerings of the area. Activities such as camping, weekend hikes, cross-country skiing, or, God forbid, snowshoeing were all on our list of "things to do as a family."

Fine. But as we grew older it took a great deal of creativity on the part of my parents, most notably my father, to keep a couple of bored teens engaged and entertained during these family outings. Of course, this was before the Internet or the bounty of digital devices available to kids these days. But like kids today, we wanted to do anything other than clomp around in nature every weekend. We wanted to be home, hanging out with our friends or just watching TV. "Another mile?" was the eternal refrain echoing through the hills.

With just a stick or a rock, our dad would invent all sorts of fun challenges on the fly that kept my brother and me entertained just long enough for an afternoon hike. Remember that phrase: "Just long enough." I mention this because sometimes we can't bog ourselves down with the big picture. Sometimes it's the moments, small valuable moments, that we're after here. Just long enough to drink an adult frosty cold one.

The activities my dad was famous for initiating on our family excursions in the wild included fort building contests, creating musical instruments, some kind of crazy sport involving pinecones, or hunting for space aliens. All these weird little things he would task us with kept us busy and happy just long enough, so he and my mom could go and "set up the tent" (nice one, Dad) or just enjoy nature.

Before my brother and I knew it, the activity he invented for us resulted in a nice pile of collected wood for the fire, or we had cleaned up all the litter left by some previous campers. Wait . . . what? How'd that happen? While we were having fun, we unwittingly helped out!?

Pretty sneaky and pretty smart.

As I grew older and began working with kids, I reflected often on these activities. I recall their important simplicity as well as the way they satisfied a moment while silently imparting larger life lessons. While they often related to a larger thesis, Dad didn't get bogged down with that. He was just trying to get through the next few minutes in relative peace.

It was the way he came up with these activities so quickly and effortlessly that always impressed me, as did how successful these simple creative activities were at keeping Shawn and me so engaged and entertained for the time required.

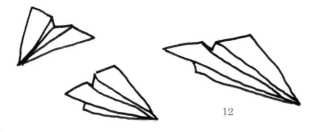

As I've developed creative programs for kids over the years, I've found myself adapting many of my dad's tricks. I've learned to use what kids themselves are bringing to the table already, their own experiences and ideas. Then like mental judo, I mesh what I want them to do with what they are interested in, then hand it back to them in the shape of an activity. Want to take something apart? Take apart this chair, then make something else. Want to throw things? Make a paper airplane and see how far you can throw it. Great things happen when your intuition meets your empathy.

WHO'S YOUR DADDY? ME, THAT'S WHO.

Now that I'm a dad, I find myself faced with keeping a couple of crazy kids engaged and entertained. Difference is I'm not coaxing them down a trail through the forest every weekend. Rather, I'm trying to get them to help out around the house, be self-reliant, and most importantly, stay off the computer and all their digital devices while trying to do my own "dad stuff."

Another difference is my situation is compounded by the fact that I'm a single dad.

Which just means the stuff I need to spend time doing has become a bit more challenging than it was before. Sure, like many of us I could use a little strengthening of my time-management skills, but even still we all could use some new tricks to keep everyone happy, healthy, and entertained.

Generally, as parents, we feel like we aren't spending enough quality time with our kids. Books and the DIY media are all too quick to offer new ways to spend more time with your kids like building go-carts in the garage or building that tree house! Don't get me wrong—spending time with your kids is always a good thing, but when we don't have 48 hours of undivided attention to offer our kids (or hundreds of dollars lying around to buy supplies), are we failures as parents?

For all of you out there stressing that the amount of time you spend with your kids isn't enough, the truth is this: Kids don't always want us on top of them telling them which screwdriver to use or how to throw a football. Sometimes they just want to do and learn along the way on their own. In most cases, kids get bored because they've tapped their shallow "idea" reserves, and they simply require new input, new ideas . . . A situation not to be interpreted by us as "come spend time with me," but rather, "give me something fun to do and go away."

It's a situation that is actually a valuable opportunity for both of you. If we stop, take a breath, and give ourselves half a second to switch up how we look at this situation, we allow ourselves to see the opportunity for what it is. This is our chance to fill their tank with new, cool, creative ideas.

So, before you ruin this teachable moment with an apology for not being your child's free, full-time entertainment system (or simply handing over the phone), look the situation right in its beady little eyes and offer something of value to make the afternoon a better and more enjoyable experience for everyone.

As I said, little moments like these can actually be special, and that's exactly the reason for this book. So, pick it up . . . oh wait, you already did. OK. Well, thumb through it and find an activity that fits your situation . . . and go for it.

Hopefully the activities in this book will get you thinking. At least that's what they're meant to do. To be perfectly clear, I'm not reinventing the wheel here, just painting it a different color.

The activities offered are not meant to provide you with a cheeky excuse to forget about your kids and pour another glass of wine for you and your enabling childless friend (that's just a bonus).

Rather, it's about thinking about your relationship with your kids in a slightly different way while, at the same time, allowing you some precious moments to get something done.

Like pouring that glass of wine.

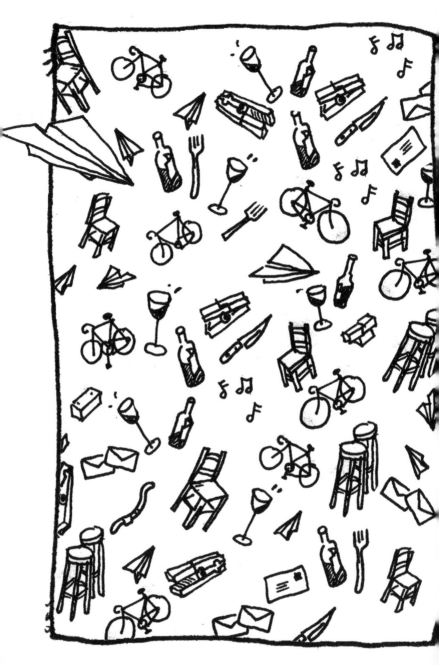

CHAPTER ONE:
CREATIVE INDOOR ACTIVITIES

From a parent's point of view, a snow day or rainy weekend can really throw a stick into the spokes of a well-planned afternoon. Of course, if this happens during the week it can be even more of a headache for anyone with kids.

While kids are giddy with joy and excitement about missing a day of school, the complete opposite is true for parents. Now it's time to figure out the kids' plan.

At this point, if you're like me and desperate, you might dial up a movie marathon for the kids to watch. It's a solid, albeit shortsighted, plan that never really works. Where you and I might love to spend the day in bed, binge watching *Arrested Development*, most kids, especially younger ones, will get bored of movies by hour two and want to move around.

At some point their little bodies will need to move! All that movie watching has just juiced up their energy level and soon they begin to vibrate and you feel they're angling toward your phone and iPads! You know that if they enter into digital device land, it'll be next to impossible to call them back. What now?

1. OLD-FASHIONED TREASURE HUNT

Keep Kids Busy For:
30–45 minutes

You Will Need:
- *2 one-dollar bills*
- *A straight face*

"There comes a time in every rightly constructed boy's life when he has a raging desire to go somewhere and dig for hidden treasure."

—Mark Twain

Throughout history, treasure hunting has captured the imagination of curious minds. Adventurers have launched expeditions to the tops of the highest peaks, to the depths of the deepest oceans, and to far-off distant lands.

The promises of long-lost treasures, kingdoms of gold, fountains of youth, and other mysteries have driven men mad and led many to early graves. But these vain efforts still inspire new generations of young hopefuls.

Even for us less adventurous we can understand the allure.

From the run-of-the-mill scavenger hunts to more traditional Easter egg hunts, we've seen 'em all. Heck, maybe you even bought one of those cheap metal detectors so the kids can dig around in the garden or the beach for lost keys or spare change. It's that mystery, that curiosity, that I've tried to capture with this activity.

Today it's your turn to kick off the next great hunt for untold treasures in your own home.

But how do you get the attention of your intended audience? Start with an introduction like this:

"That's right!" you say with great flourish to a room of kids staring motionless at another episode of *Wizards of Waverly Place.* "There is adventure afoot!" Now, if the television program's canned laughter is the only response to your exciting declaration, have no fear. Pull out the big guns. "Somewhere in this room I hid three single dollar bills and you have forty-five minutes to find them!" Wait for it . . . "And if you find them, you can keep them!" Now they heard you!

Quickly in one seamless, fluid motion, switch off the screen and lay down the rules.

As they are in most activities, rules are key to the enjoyment. For this activity, they're pretty simple and you can adjust as needed.

First, if it's nice outside and you want to kick the kids out of the house for a couple of hours, this would be a great activity to get them moving in that direction. If you do end up conducting this activity outside, stick with a specific area that will keep the kids from wandering the neighborhood looking for the hidden money. Your neighbors might start to talk.

Back to the *booty*; it's important not to hide the treasure too well. If you really hide it, the kids will get tired of looking and your incessant laughter will only make them more frustrated and ready to quit. You can be sure if that happens it'll be the last treasure hunt you'll ever be allowed to host. On the flip side, if it's too easy, it's like you're giving money away, and who wants that? Try to hide the treasure just well enough that you can count on some quality time by yourself. Keep in mind, you're *paying* for this time.

As for the actual treasure, you can hide any equivalent and in any denomination you'd like. Just don't hide enough for everyone to find something. It might seem mean hearted, but kids don't learn from winning, they learn the big lessons from losing in most cases. I know that's not politically correct to say, especially coming from me sitting here in Berkeley, California, but it's true, and this activity is no different. Let 'em lose!

Here's why having some kids not finding the treasure is important: When the game is over the losers will pressure the winners into hiding their rewards again for another round . . . duh! Then you get two or maybe even three games, literally, for the price of one. And when the final round is reached, you'll realize that real money isn't even the point anymore. It was just a tool to get the kids interested in doing something *real*!

Lastly, don't let the kids ask you any questions, and don't give them any hints. That'll be the first thing they ask. "Do we get any hints?" or "Will you tell us if we're getting warmer?"

"Sorry kids. That's a big negative on both counts. No hints and no temperature gauge! You guys are on your own. Next time I see you, it should be when somebody wins. Got it? Good. I'll be inside/in the other room working. Good luck."

Which brings me to the next bit to remember. Let them know this is a one-time shot kinda game. You're only hiding X amount of dollars once and unless the winner wants to throw their winnings back into play, it's over. For your own good, don't be a pushover. It could get expensive!

ADDED NOTE: There is a dark-ish side to the treasure hunt activity. I'd like to offer this version to those among us without the burden of scruples who find themselves in dire straights. It's simple. Just *tell* the kids you hid some money in the backyard. Don't actually do it of course. The amount doesn't matter. Just tell the kids it's out there and whoever finds it, can keep it! Bam. Done. All that's left to do is prop open the door.

When the kids come back in winded and frustrated 30 or so minutes later, asking for the exact whereabouts of the phantom treasure, or at least a hint, you can just shrug and say, "Sorry kids. If you can't find it, I'll have to go out later and get it and no one wins!" A cheap ploy to be sure, but effective.

WARNING: *Try to concentrate the activity to a certain area to keep the kids from getting off track and wandering away from the intended game site.*

HINT: *Don't hide enough treasure so that everyone can find something. Losers can be key in pressuring the winners to hide their treasure again for another round.*

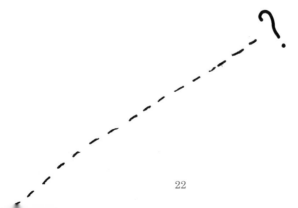

2. AN ALL-AMERICAN JUNK DRAWER CHALLENGE

Keep Kids Busy For:
30–45 minutes

You Will Need:
One unorganized junk drawer

Having one or two junk drawers in your home is an important part of what we all consider to be key characteristics of the great American household. It's that go-to place where we're sure to find all our pens, paper clips, lost game pieces tucked beneath old maps, and old forgotten refrigerator magnets.

A perfect place where all the odds and ends we encounter in our lives get deposited and are always accessible. Yes, it's the junk drawer that keeps America from really losing its proverbial mind.

So, you got your junk drawer, but did you know that in every junk drawer there's an adventure just waiting for someone willing to take the time to sort through it? Well, there is! And this is an activity just perfect for little hands to explore and discover.

But before we go any further, do yourself a favor and take a second to quickly go through the contents prior to allowing those little hands access. I don't know about you, but I would not want my me-time interrupted with questions like "Daddy, what's this for?" or "Daddy, is this yours?" Also don't forget to remove any sharp objects. We wouldn't want any blood in the drawer.

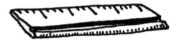

To begin this activity, pull the drawer of junk completely out and off the track, placing it on a flat surface, like a table or the floor. Now it's time to construct the adventure.

Asking the kids a question or giving them a challenge is a perfect motivation to get the adventure started, but coming up with good ideas can be tricky. You want to make it fun and kind of challenging, but if you make your challenges too challenging, the kids will get bored and just ask to play on your phone.

Try and come up with challenges that are age appropriate and just subjective enough to keep them engaged for at least 20–30 minutes. **Try these to get started:**

1. Try and connect as many things in the drawer together to create a tower as high as you can.

2. Create faces by laying out the items on the table. What would make a good mouth, or what would be good to use for hair?

3. Color-code everything in the drawer like a rainbow.

4. Organize the junk in the drawer any way that you would like.

5. Count all the change . . . and figure your 10 percent cut.

Another great activity based around the contents of the drawer is to have the kids make up a story based on twelve random things they find in the drawer! After they figure it out they have to tell you the story.

The brilliant thing about junk drawer adventures is that you get way more out of the whole thing than the kids do, to be honest. Sure they have fun exploring the contents of the mystery drawer, but if you play your cards well you could get a clean and organized drawer out of the deal! And, most importantly, you get some time to yourself. That's what is commonly referred to as a "win-win"!

WARNING: *Remember: Remove all sharp and incriminating objects from the drawer before letting any little hands explore the contents.*

HINT: *Have a few age-appropriate challenges ready before you begin just in case one doesn't work.*

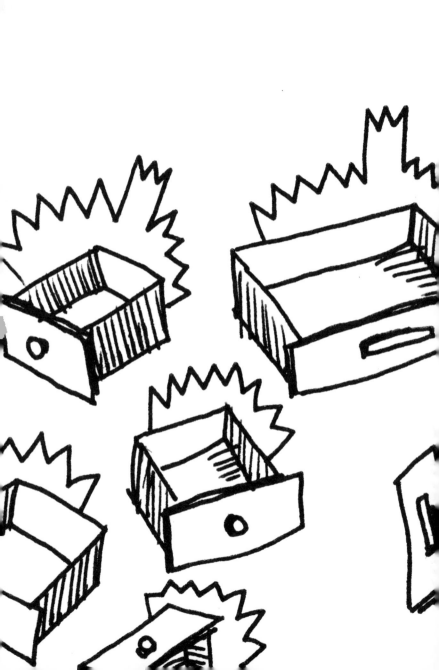

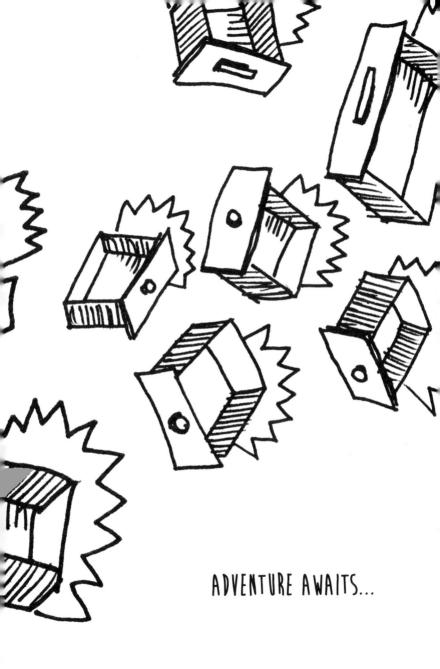

ADVENTURE AWAITS...

3. Occupy the Living Room
(A.K.A. Fort City)

Keep Kids Busy For:
120+ minutes

You Will Need:
- *Blankets*
- *Pillows*
- *Flashlights*
- *Other assorted and approved household items*

It always makes activities a more fun and effective teaching moment when you can tie current or recent events into the activities you offer your kids. It helps in making the experience a tad more educational. Plus, any kids you may be hosting for the afternoon will go home and recount the activity to their parents and you'll get superior cool-cred for being so hip and informed. Which is important. #justsaying

This activity is of course based on the Occupy movement that swept the nation not too long ago. It introduced a new generation to the power of a good protest.

Now, it also serves to freshen up that traditional childhood activity of building a blanket tent inside the house!

Occupy the Living Room!

I don't know a kid out there who would turn down a chance to build a tent in the living room. Even my thirteen-year-old likes to do this. I mean, building a tent fort in their own room is fun and all, but being given the chance to take over the common space of the home is like getting the keys to the city! Tent city!

To begin this particular activity, I suggest collecting all the appropriate blankets you have lying around, such as the ones on their beds, and maybe throw in a couple towels and tablecloths, if you have them, as well. Once you collect this stuff, place it neatly in the middle of the living room floor. At this point you could also drag a chair in from the kitchen and maybe a broom to help hold up any saggy parts. You doing all this should get them interested enough to ask a couple of questions such as, "What are you doing?" or "Why are you putting all that stuff in here?" But you say nothing at first. After you've assembled everything you can tell them your idea while you are actually beginning to build the tent.

Begin by draping one end over that chair you brought in from the kitchen, the other end tucked under a cushion of the couch, lay out some cushions for some interior walls, and so on. Soon the kids will just have to jump in and show you how to really build a blanket tent.

At this point you back away feigning ignorance and leave them to it. Got 'em!

But as you're slowly backing away and angling back to your laptop and your 11 a.m. glass of wine, leave them with a couple of well-chosen rules. **I suggest the following:**

1. They have to move any furniture back to the way it was when they're done.

2. Anyone who helps to build it must help to clean it up. (This locks in any of the kids' friends who might decide to go home before any clean-up is required.)

3. No lights other than flashlights can be used. (Potential fire hazard there.)

4. No other blankets can be used. (This keeps the kids from stripping your bed and the remaining sheets off their own beds.)

Then, when it's finally time for friends to go home and the tent city to come down, just as in real life, prepare yourself for that traditional chant of the dispossessed: "Hell no, we won't go! Hell no, we won't go!" Good luck there!

WARNING: *Of course there are a couple of things to remember when allowing your kids and their friends to begin construction on a tent city in the living room. First, you should probably remove fragile items from the area, as these* *will break! Pointy things should also be removed, as these will inflict pain and/or wounds. Nothing puts a damper on a well-constructed afternoon like cleaning up blood.*

HINT: *To give this particular activity some traction, tell the kids that you intend to visit the encampment in 45 minutes and that everything should be set up and ready for visitors. Including some individual rooms built out. When the 45-minute mark is reached, go visit and tell them that you will return again in 30 minutes with popcorn. By setting these time increments they will continue to build and expand on the structure wanting to impress you. Plus, you'll get some time to check your email and such.*

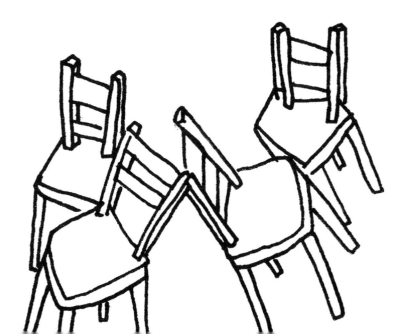

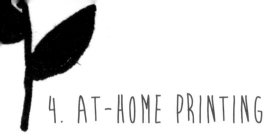

4. AT-HOME PRINTING

Keep Kids Busy For:
45–60 minutes

You Will Need:
- *Acrylic paint (different colors)*
- *Cookie sheet*
- *Large paintbrush*
- *Thin paintbrush*
- *Drop cloth (or newspaper to cover the flat work space)*
- *Pencil (with eraser)*
- *Paper (card stock or any heavy paper)*
- *Rolling pin*
- *Various household items for texture*

Printing is a fun way for the kids to roll up their sleeves and get a little messy! The pictures they make will be perfect for framing, greeting cards, or even wrapping paper.

This is craftier than most of the other activities in this book, but still it's a great way to reuse a bunch of stuff lying around the house.

There are a couple of different kinds of printing techniques that I'll introduce in this section which are perfect to try at home. They're easy, you can let the kids do them without you having to hover over them too much, and they're easy to clean up too . . . especially if you have a little table outside and the weather is cooperating.

EASY MONO PRINTING

"Mono" printing is a form of printmaking where you're only making one print at a time, unlike other types of printmaking where you're making multiple originals. The simple version of this technique is fun and easy and you can use anything you might find around the house. Assemble items like a little dirt, keys, or anything else that can lie on the paint to make an interesting pattern or texture on your paper.

To get started, turn your cookie sheet upside down and apply a thin (but not too thin) layer of paint with your large brush directly onto the bottom of your cookie sheet. Use the bottom of the cookie sheet so you don't have to mind the lip of the sheet.

For best results, make the spread of paint slightly smaller than the full surface you plan to print on. Once the paint has been applied, you can also let the kids draw in the paint using their fingers or the eraser end of the pencil. You can leave the drawing as the print or add objects like the keys to the design.

Once the design is complete you're ready to make a print!

To print, lay the paper you want to print on top of the painted surface and lightly rub with the heel of your palm or roll the surface with a rolling pin evenly and slowly with just slight pressure.

Roll or rub the full area to be printed, making sure to get even contact for best results. Be careful when rubbing or rolling your print so you don't move or smudge the design. If keeping your paper in place while transferring is difficult, try taping the paper in place before rubbing.

After a couple of minutes, gently lift the paper off the paint and check your print. If it doesn't come out as you had hoped, don't get discouraged. It might take a few times to get comfortable with the process. Sometimes the little mistakes or inconsistencies are what make printing this way fun and unique!

If the kids are feeling a little experimental, they could try laying paper shapes onto their painted design to block out the paint on their paper, allowing spaces for you to write into later. It's perfect for invitations or thank-you notes. There are tons of fun things to do with this kind of printing.

After some practice, you will begin to get an idea of the process and become more comfortable. Be mindful about how much paint is needed, how hard and how long you need to rub before you lift the paper, and what kind of things work best to make cool shapes come out.

BLOCK PRINTING

You've heard of potato prints. This is just like that, except I'm also including anything with a good and pronounced texture, like Legos, tree bark, or even hands. We can really use anything that has an interesting texture with enough relief that it'll make a print after being dipped in paint and pressed onto a surface.

To get started, go on a little expedition around the house to find possible items before you get everyone's attention. Searching for appropriate items to be dipped in paint is your job and not something you want the kids to do on their own for obvious reasons, especially if they're little. Grab a couple of old veggies from the bin of your refrigerator, a handful of stale pretzels, a swatch or two of some fibrous cloth like burlap, and a couple of keys, and you'll be ready to go!

One of the great things about printing this way is you can really use almost anything you might have lying around. Anything from crumpled pieces of paper to old vegetables. Got some cardboard TP tubes? Rolled-up newspapers? Soda cans? Really anything that will leave some kind of impression will be perfect for this activity. But be prepared . . . while getting your kids ready to do this, you might actually get into it too and start making your own prints! Then your free time goes out the window and time with your kids comes into play. But don't get me wrong, that kind of time is well spent too. It's just not what this book is about. Now, for making the mark you can really use anything from food dyes to India ink to some kinds of paint. Dip one of the objects into your paint or ink, then onto some laid-out paper or some previously OK'd clothes, and presto, you've got cool new designs. Make sure you're letting your fresh work dry before throwing it in the wash or putting it on. Above all, make sure you used fabric paint for clothing.

Like I said before, the actual term for this kind of printing is mono-printing, meaning you make only one rather than repeating the process to make dozens by reapplying paint or ink.

WARNING: *Paint and ink can, and will probably, stain. So make sure you and the kids are properly dressed for this activity and your surface is covered! It also helps to use paint and nontoxic, nonstaining paint and inks. Either way a suitable work space with plenty of fresh air is a perfect spot to get into this. Remember to work quickly before the paint begins to dry. Also, when doing the mono-printing, don't use things that are too thick or big when making your print, as it will keep the paper from making contact with the paint.*

HINT: *Before laying your paper down on the surface to be printed, you may want to try wetting it first ever so slightly* *to help give the paper a little more looseness in its grain. This will allow it to more easily lie down and pick up all the details, especially for mono-printing. The slight dampness also helps to transfer the paint to the paper.*

Use some of the work the kids produce to offer an alternative to the tired lemonade stand! Have a front yard art sale instead! (see Pop-Up Art Stand, p 156) *Make designs suitable for framing and throw together a quick art sale in the front yard with their friends.*

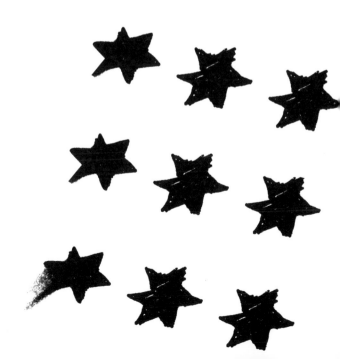

5. PLAY-WITH DOUGH

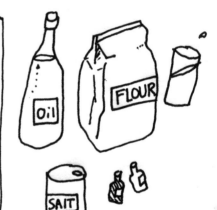

Keep Kids Busy For:
30–45 minutes

You Will Need:
- *Water*
- *Flour*
- *Vegetable oil*
- *Salt*
- *Food coloring*
- *Saucepan*
- *Bowl*

We all had this crap as kids. You know, that weird molding compound available in primary colors and packed in those little plastic buckets with lids.

That strange claylike material actually began as wallpaper cleaner back in the 1950s—I kid you not. I don't remember playing with the stuff as much as just smelling it. I loved the way it smelled. Now of course you can go out and purchase this dough whenever you want, but why? Especially after I tell you how crazy easy it is to make at home, and making it is half the fun.

Here's how to make your own nontoxic Play-With Dough! If you go and search out dough recipes on the web, you'll find two different types out there: cooked and uncooked.

I prefer the cooked kind because it has a better texture and feels better in the hand than the uncooked kind. Of course, since there is a stove-top involved, you'll have to locate yourself nearby if you're letting the kids make this.

The basic ingredients for my favorite Play-With Dough:

*2 **cups** basic white flour*

*2 **cups** warm water*

*1 **cup** table salt*

*2 **tablespoons** vegetable oil*

*1 **tablespoon** cream of tartar*

For colors, you can use food coloring.

Mix all of the ingredients together (except food coloring), and stir the mix over a very low heat until your dough begins to thicken.

When the dough begins to resemble thick bread dough, pulling away from the sides of the pan, and starts clumping in the center of the pan, remove from the heat and let cool. If your Play-With Dough is still sticky, continue to stir over low heat until you get the right consistency. When the dough is cool, you can add in a couple of drops of the coloring of your choice and work the color in with your hands until it's even and awesome.

WARNING: *Fight the urge to eat the dough or feed it to your pets. There's a lot of salt in the dough and that is not good for you or your pets!*

HINT: *Double the recipe and put some in a plastic bag for another day. When applying the color, try separating your dough out and using a few different colors rather than just one. I like making some dough blue, some red, and a little green.*

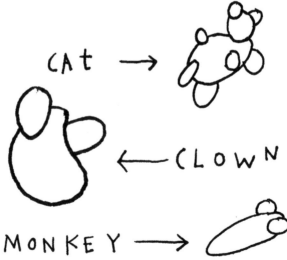

6. APOCALYPSE BUTTER CANDLES

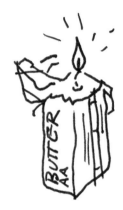

Keep Kids Busy For:
30 minutes

You Will Need:
- *1 Stick of cold butter*
- *Toilet tissue*
- *Matches*
- *Butter knife*
- *Plate or piece of foil*

File this activity under: "Just in case of zombie apocalypse." Making candles is about as crafty as you can get. Nothing says "über-crafty hipster" more than standing over your kitchen sink making candles. If that might be a worry of yours, let me assure you right off the bat, these are no ordinary candles! These are butter candles! Butter candles? Yes, butter candles.

Really, butter is not such a strange material to use for candles. As you may recall, back in the day, candles were made from the rendered fat from various animals. In fact, rendering whale fat was used in the earliest known candles by the Chinese, during the Qin Dynasty, 221–206 BC. So it kind of figures that butter would work in a similar "fatty" sorta way. And it does.

The first thing you're going to want to do is have the kids take out a single paper-wrapped stick of butter and unwrap one end just to expose the end of the butter. Once the end of the butter is exposed, take a sharp pencil and poke about a ¼-inch hole into the end of the butter. This is where you're going to bury one end of the "wick."

To make the wick, take a single square of toilet tissue and twist it, rolling it into a long thin worm. Once you have the length tightly wound, stick one end into the hole you made with the pencil. Once it's in, close the butter hole around the wick, getting butter all over the entire wick as you go.

At this point you should have a stick of butter still wrapped in paper except the end. In the exposed end of your butter you should have a "wick" of toilet tissue sticking out. It should look like a candle or a greasy butter-shaped explosive.

Now all that's left to do is to place your candle on a plate or a piece of foil and light 'er up! You'll be surprised how long it will stay lit!

WARNING: *This is an easy process, but try and do it quickly so the butter doesn't melt on you. Also keep any eye on it and* watch the paper wrapper on the stick so that it doesn't burn. It shouldn't, but that doesn't mean it won't. As with any candle, don't light it up and leave the room for any extended period of time.

HINT: *When you put the wick into the end of the butter stick, make sure to get the exposed wick lightly covered in butter. This will feed the flame and keep the tissue paper from burning completely up as tissue would normally.*

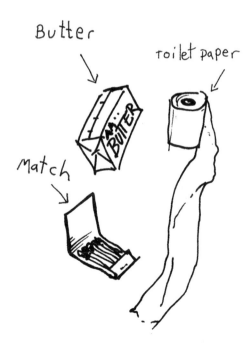

7. PEBBLE PEOPLE

> **Keep Your Kids Busy For:**
> *30–45 minutes*
>
> **You Will Need:**
> - *10–15 Smooth stones*
> - *Colored markers*
> - *Paper*

Sometimes you don't have a bunch of fancy materials on hand to keep the kids entertained. I know that a lot of the crafty books for parents out there just assume we all have a well-appointed craft pantry ready and stocked for any project that comes to mind. They also seem to think we all have unlimited free time to sit down with little Billy and little Susie and cut out clouds . . . or would even want to.

This is reality folks. It's flooding outside, the kids are home from school, you're "working" from home, and you need to get the kids off the computer so you can join a Skype meeting that started about 10 minutes ago. Ugh.

You might not know it, but you need the help of Pebble People! (a.k.a. something you can get the kids started on and leave them for a good amount of time while you save your job.)

We've all heard of pet rocks, right? Ever think about the rock families that those pet rocks belonged to? I have, and to get this activity started, I suggest you do too.

"Hey kids, run outside and grab some pebbles and small smooth rocks. I've got a plan." While they're out there, quickly grab some markers and pens and lay them out on a table with a few sheets of blank paper from the printer.

When the kids come back in, clean and dry off the rocks and put them on the table with the pens and paper. Have the kids gather 'round and take a good long look at each of their rocks and see if they can *find* a face. Ask them, "What kind of face is it? Happy? Sad?" Once they see those little rock faces then they can take a pen and a marker and make that face more visible, and give their Pebble People names.

At the end, they should have transformed the small rocks into cute little heads with amusing little faces with their own little expressions! But what about the paper, how is that used? Good question.

After the kids have created their Pebble People, they can continue the activity by designing little environments on the paper to place their Pebble People on. They can draw rooms and houses where their Pebble People might live, and maybe even create a little hike for their Pebbles to follow through mountains or cities. You could even grab some dice so they can make a game using the Pebble People as pieces to move along the game route! Gosh dang I'm good.

Pebble People are surprisingly versatile and well traveled. They can do anything. They can live next to kids' beds, sit and watch over plants, be cute little surprises in drawers and cupboards, and more. Pebble People fit into pockets and backpacks, they live in pools or on dashboards.
Pebble People can go anywhere—trains, planes, or even boats! Basically Pebble People are awesome. Yay. Good luck with your meeting.

WARNING: *Pebble People DO NOT fly. I repeat, Pebble People DO NOT fly.*

HINT: *Don't use any rocks larger than the kids' fist for this activity. Keep it to small smooth stones for best results!*

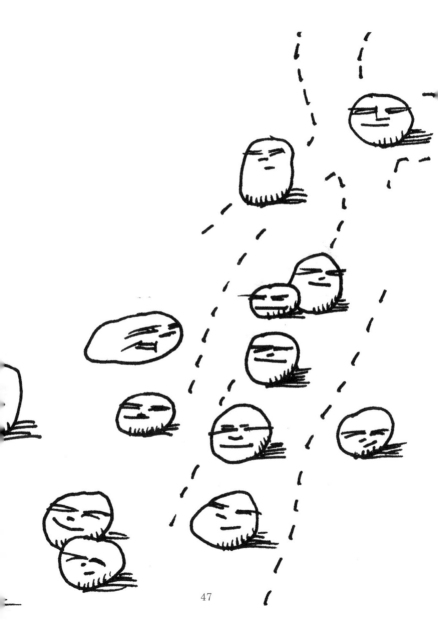

8. FISTFUL O' COINS

How many coins do you think you could hold in one hand? 30? 50? Now, how much monetary value do you think you have there? 2 bucks? Maybe 4? Maybe it's all pennies and you have just 40 cents!

The basic idea here is twofold; First, how many coins can you grab with one hand? And second, how much value can you grab with one hand? You can hold fewer coins and have more value than someone with a huge fist full of coins that could be all pennies.

That's what this game is all about. Your big hairy adult hands aren't going to help you secure the big win this time. There is a lovely amount of luck involved here, which means

your kids could beat you. But why are you playing anyway? Don't you have to go *check your email*? or *take out
the garbage*? Get the kids set up and leave them alone.

Obviously, you need a pretty healthy amount of coins to
play with. So go bust out the big coin jar you have in the
closet, grab some paper, a pencil, and call the kids. You
have something really important to share with them.

Depending on the age of the kids in your charge for the
afternoon, you might want to jot down the value of each
coin on a separate slip of paper for the younger ones to
refer to so they don't keep running to you asking how
much they have.

Let's get started.

The best way to do this is to simply dump all the coins
into a pillowcase and let each player reach in and grab
a fistful of coins. No long periods of "rooting" around
here. We want to use a simple "grab-n-go" technique.
After grabbing a fistful-o-coins, each child empties
their hand onto a clear section of the floor or table for
counting. Count how many coins and how much value
in each grab.

It's important that one person goes at a time, since
you'll need to return the "grabbed" coins back into the
sack. That way everyone has all the original amount of

coins to grab from, plus everyone can pitch in and help with the scoring.

For keeping score, you'll need two columns for each player. The first column is for the "amount" or how many coins in each hand, and the second column for the "value" of each hand. If you want to add a third column, you could write down specifically how many pennies, and how many nickels, etc. are in the "grab." . . . That's up to you and the kind of game you want to play.

Once everyone has a go, total up the columns and see who comes out ahead. The way this activity is set up, you could actually have two or more winners. I say that for the benefit of those of you who happen to be parents or guardians who need everyone to "win." Don't get me started on this. Let me just say that you can't have a winner without having a loser. Just saying. I mean, if you can't allow kids to fail or lose every once in a while then they'll never learn to try harder. So, I urge you all out there to allow your kids to fall, get hurt, fail, or lose. Start now. Thank me later. Good luck.

WARNING: *Some kids might feel left out if they aren't confident with their math skills or their knowledge of coin values yet. Make a quick and easy cheat sheet for the whole group to refer to during the game.*

HINT: *It's always a good idea to clean the coins, but if you don't, or can't, clean them first, it's not a bad idea to have some wet wipes or hand sanitizer nearby. Money is dirty.*

	DAD	ROMY
Pennies	48 = $.48	15 = $.15
Nickels	17 = $.60	10 = $.50
Dimes	16 = $1.60	19 = $1.90
Quarters	3 = $.75	6 = $1.50
	$3.43	$4.05

9. SHADOW PUPPETS

Keep Kids Busy For:
30–60 minutes

You Will Need:
- *Some string*
- *Egg carton*
- *Desk lamp*

Shadows can be awesome for any kid to play with. And no, I'm not being facetious. I've used shadows in many of my workshops for kids and adults. In fact, shadows are just another material like anything else. Creating something that will cast an interesting shadow means thinking about objects in a slightly different way than we usually do. Usually, we work and think with the positive form or mass like a sculpture. But when we turn that slightly on its side and think about the negative, the reaction, the effect our positive form casts, we actually see an extension, a new idea.

It makes a nice metaphor, which is why it makes for such a great workshop or part of a memorable class project. When dealing with the shadow of something, we don't get three dimensions, we only get a rough estimation of size and angle. It's actually a lot like stenciling. You aren't just working with light you allow, but also the light you don't allow.

Where do we begin with this? Sure, we've all tried making animals or people with your hands on the bedroom wall. You might rock the shadow puppet, but for me, they all look like a fist and I end up with a hand cramp. So thankfully, the difference here is that instead of just hands, try using a shoebox or any other simple materials like string. With a shoebox we can create many little sculptures or one big one that throws cool, interesting shadows on the wall or even on the ground outside.

You could also do this outside if you have some sun, but if you're stuck inside because of un-sunny weather you can use a desk lamp against a bedroom wall.

When using only one piece of material, you've gotta give the kids something more to work with. So in this case, come up with a subject or a storyline for the kids to expand on. Stuff like "Traveling Across the Sea" or "Hunting for Big Game in the Wild Jungle" are good ones. Games are always better and more imaginative if you frame them like book titles. That way, the kids will be more naturally inclined to come up with a story to go along with your title. You could also use actual titles of books they may be reading, like *Where the Wild Things Are*, and ask them to act out the stories.

Besides exploring a new dimension of materiality, you're throwing in a little science as well. On the science front, kids will quickly realize that the shadows cast by using a desk lamp inside are quite different than manipulating their sculptures outside in the sunlight. Why is that? They can play with the size of their shadows by getting closer to or farther away from the light source inside, but can they do that outside? How does the sun's angle affect form?

If you can get the kids to stop looking at the thing in their hands and only look at the shadow, they may notice the form they're holding in their hands might look odd and completely different from what they see in the shadow. This is very fun, thought-provoking stuff to play with. And who knows, maybe you'll discover you have a junior scientist on your hands.

The final part to this activity could be a multimedia presentation if you'd like to let your kids borrow your phone, or God forbid, they have one of their own. Ask them to make a shadow movie, or take some pictures for a gallery show.

The kids have to make it happen with just the egg carton and string. If you trust your kids with your phone or a video camera, it might be a good opportunity for them to make a little movie . . . or not. Actually, you know what? Scrap that idea, don't give them your phone. That's just asking for trouble!

WARNING: *Keep an eye on how the kids are arranging the lamps in attempts to get the perfect shadow. It's all good fun, but lamps can start fires.*

HINT: *Give your kids a few different pieces of materials to play with. Egg cartons, string, plastic bags, or bits of cloth are all good things to have on hand when making shadows.*

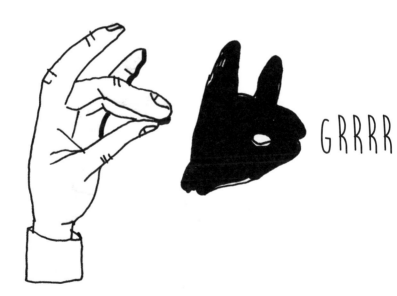

GRRRR

10. PAPER AIRPLANES

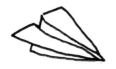

The true test of one's mettle has and will always be measured by how well one can fold and fly a simple paper airplane. It's a fact. I know it sounds crazy, but think about it. If you can't fold a moderately successful paper airplane, you might as well give up.

But you say you want to learn? Well then. Paper airplanes are great for kids, especially if there's a competition! How far can yours go? Can yours do tricks? A couple of seconds on the web will result in literally hundreds of videos and images of different paper airplanes and how to fold them. Some of the best, farthest-flying paper airplanes don't even look like airplanes at all!

Of all the options out there, the basic is the "Dart." The Dart is a simple and probably the most well-known paper airplane. It's easy to fold, and flies fast and far. The Dart is also easy to manipulate. With little folds and some straightening here and there, you can make the plane soar up or soar low, twist, and turn.

Grab a few sheets of paper and let's give this one a try, going step by step. Remember, as in life, the first folds are the most important to get right. Fold clean, even, and straight.

Step 1. *First fold your 8.5" x 11" piece of paper in half lengthwise and run your thumbnail along the fold. Doing that helps to crease it sharply and cleanly. Then unfold the paper flat.*

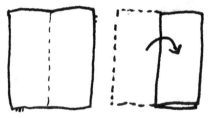

Step 2. *Fold down the top corners, so that the top corners meet along the center fold line.*

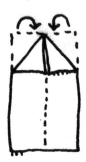

Step 3. *Fold the two sides of the paper so they meet at that center fold line.*

Step 4. *Make a kind of "valley" fold in half. Then turn the plane 90 degrees.*

Step 5. *Create a wing by making a crease beginning at the nose.*

Step 6. *Ta-Da! Your Dart is complete.*
Play around with bending the tail edges of the wings to create more lift if your dart keeps nose-diving.

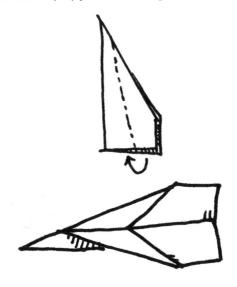

WARNING: *Make sure you have plenty of letter size (8.5" x 11") paper on hand before getting started. This activity can go through a lot of paper.*

HINT: *Kids might be more inclined to give their all if there's an airplane contest. When everyone has their planes constructed, try a contest measuring the distance the planes can fly.*

11. YOU COMPLETE ME (THEE EXQUISITE CORPSE)

Keep Kids Busy For:
30–45 minutes

You Will Need:
- *Pen and paper (lined and /or unlined)*
- *An odd sense of humor*

As a Gothy, artistic teen in high school, I used to love the name of this activity: "Thee Exquisite Corpse." OK. I added the "thee" for Shakespearian effect. But even without my help, it still sounds ghoulish, and so Edward Gorey! You pass a sheet of paper around, inviting everyone to add a little piece of inspiration and see what is created at the end.

Before we get started, let's get into a little of the history and origin of this mysterious and fun indoor activity.

"Exquisite Corpse" was developed around 1925 as an artistic exercise by French surrealist writer André Breton, who started it initially as a fun game to play when his cheap artist friends came around and drank copious amounts of his absinthe and smoked all of his lovely French cigarettes. (Not so, here. Daddy will be keeping his absinthe and Gauloises for himself and any fancy French friends he meets.)

In French, the game was originally termed *cadavre exquis* meaning "exquisite cadaver" or "rotating corpse." Essentially, it's a method by which participants collect words or images, taking turns and adding to a composition a.k.a. the corpse. This is done either by having everyone follow some literary rule or just by being allowed to see only the very end of what the previous person contributed, such as the last sentence someone wrote, or the last little bit of what the previous person drew.

The technique, according to Breton, was started just for fun, but soon became popular among his surrealist artist and writer friends. Later the game was adapted for all sorts of things like toys and children's books that we've all seen. You know the ones, where the pages were cut into thirds. The top part of the pages would show a head of a person or animal, the middle part might show a torso, and the bottom part would have legs. And kids can mix and match by turning pages and making up different combinations. We have the French surrealists to thank for those.

For this game, it's the surprise at the end we're after! Seeing what everyone wrote or drew and how they fit together is the fun part!

OK. So, now that we all know more or less what we're talking about, I'm going to propose that we change it up a bit. Since you have two, three, or even more kids doing this, we don't want them waiting around to get a turn. So, I propose each kid starts one, either by writing or drawing. We then set a timer to go off in five-minute increments, and when the buzzer goes off, the kids pass their corpse to the left. This continues for six to ten 5-minute increments.

You can give them a rule to follow like giving the whole group a category like "People" or "Animals." This will keep the work contained a bit while still being free and open to interpretation. Remember, these are kids, not French surrealists, dang it! All the same, you're taking on their horrible ennui and solving their existential crises—for the moment, anyway.

Now pass out black pens and 8.5" x 11" sheets of white paper to everyone. Ask the kids to fold their paper into thirds.

They will all begin drawing on the top third halves for 5 minutes. Once the 5 minutes are up, they fold their papers to only show the last little bits of what they wrote or drew. For example, if the first kid drew a head, pass the paper to the next kid with just the last lines of the neck showing. Each kid takes the folded paper passed to them and begins to draw or write their contribution. No looking at what the previous person passes to you!

Each "round" or page will take about 15 minutes to complete. But if each kid starts at the same time, all the crazy drawings will be finished around the same time and every kid will be busy drawing and constantly thinking of what to draw next.

WARNING: *It might be tempting to break out the absinthe and cigarettes, but kids are too young to drink or even smoke yet. So save them, or enjoy them yourself outside while the kids are busy. Better yet, when the kids go to sleep, invite your arty friends over and get a couple of adult rounds in yourself.*

HINT: *You can get the mood going by playing a little Edith Piaf on the phonograph in homage to our dear friend Breton! Also, it's important for each kid to make lines where the next kid picks up the picture. That way each contribution connects. Remember, no peeking!*

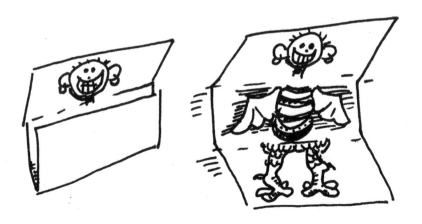

12. CLOTHESPIN TOWERS

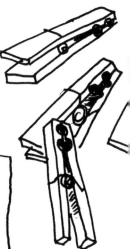

> **Keep Kids Busy For:**
> *30–45 minutes*
>
> **You Will Need:**
> * *Spring-loaded wooden clothespins*
> * *Yardstick or measuring tool*

As you probably know by now, some of the coolest, most fun toys aren't actually toys at all. At least they weren't meant to be toys!

Take clothespins for example. Not the plastic molded ones, but the wooden ones with springs that you squeeze open to attach. These things are ingenious little contraptions that make an amazing and inexpensive toy for kids of all ages. Which is a great reason to have a few bags of these on hand.

These cheaply designed spring-type clothespins were first manufactured in 1853 by David Smith, an inventor in Springfield, Vermont. He developed the wooden clothespin by creating two interlocking flat wooden pieces, with a small spring between the two. When the two prongs are pinched the prongs open up, and when released, the prongs shut. Sounds simple enough.

Quite the invention. Of course not only did it revolution-ize the hanging of laundry on a line, but Mr. Smith also unwittingly set the modern craft world ablaze.

Today there are all sorts of colorful, crafty clothespins out there to buy, but the cool ones are still the tradition-al, natural wooden ones with the metal springs that Mr. Smith developed.

You can usually find bags of fifty or so for under $5.00. Keep a couple of bags on hand, and you'll be set. Then when push comes to shove, you can throw a bag of these into the ring for your kids and you'll be happy you had them!

In my experience, when kids are offered a chance to ex-plore a material that they don't usually get to play with, they will be drawn to it like moths to a flame. Now pair that sense of curiosity with a couple of very easy direc-tives, and you should be able to keep your little ones entertained for a good amount of the afternoon.

As you may or may not know, there's a lot you can do with fifty clothespins. Heck, a couple of minutes and a web browser will yield hundreds, perhaps thousands, of fancy little craft ideas from puppets to lamp shades that are made, in some cases, entirely of clothespins. But, that's not the road we want to go down. We want some straight-up raw creativity here and next to no directions to follow.

Of course I say that, but when you introduce the bag of clothespins, it's best to have a challenge or some kind of directive to go with it. Nothing too instructional, just a broad big picture idea to get them started. It's the difference between a couple of ho-hum minutes versus a couple of hours of concentrated play.

Remember, as I said, keep your challenge subjective enough for it not to come across being too instructional that they can't experiment. But at the same time, you don't want it to be so subjective and open-ended that it's a free-for-all. Crafting the perfect challenge could be a challenge in itself.

Try this: "Hey guys, how tall can you build a tower with these?"

Then try a harmless follow-up such as, "I've got some popsicles for you in the freezer if you can build a tower with all fifty clothespins!" Then of course, just walk away.

That challenge has just enough open-endedness and just enough instruction to put the kids on a path toward something. Of course, promises of popsicles can do the trick! But I think that kids will have enough fun doing this project that you won't need to give out any treats or enticements to get them engaged.

Don't worry, there is a little trick to getting a successful tower built. That trick being: you have to taper the base in an Eiffel Tower–type shape. Architecture 101.

A wide base that narrows toward the top will increase the likelihood you will be able to get all fifty pins attached and the structure will stand solidly. Again, if you get that base solid you can easily pile on the rest of the bag on top and get some real height.

Now that you know that trick, you can swing by and offer a few handy tips to encourage the inspiration. Maybe even toss an extra bag or two of clothespins to see just how high they can go! Good luck.

WARNING: *Clothespins are fun, but try not to get too involved with the kids. Remember you have emails to go through and dinner to make. Right?*

HINT: *Keeping a few bags of these on hand is always a good idea. They're great for simple life hacks like keeping chip bags closed or clipping notes to things. Basically having a mess of these things around is better than not having them around.*

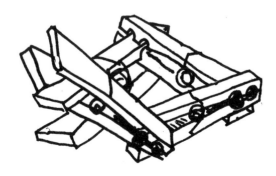

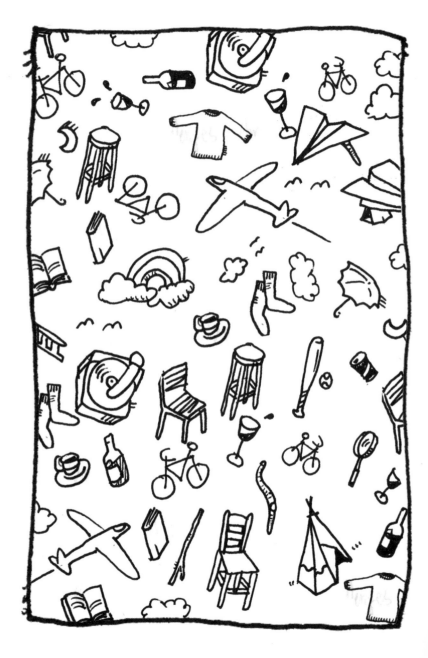

CHAPTER TWO:
KIDS EARN THEIR KEEP

The thing that gets me the most about kids these days is, they just don't seem to understand why they should have to help out around the house. It's not enough that they live, sleep, and eat here. Heck, they even invite friends to come over. But still, for some reason, the simple act of lifting a finger to clean a dish or get their dad a frosty malt beverage from the fridge *and* open it is too much of an inconvenience. The little ingrates!

That's when I resort to a little tried-and-true, admittedly underhanded trickery to get certain tasks done.

Sometimes, as I said earlier, straight-up tricking kids into doing the right thing is what's called for. Plus, you'll feel like a boss.

There are loads of little chores around the house that can easily be done by kids. But if you're like me, in most cases, it's just easier to do it yourself. At least you know it's getting done right and you don't have to explain the whole thing over and over.

For the longest time, having my kids help out around the house seemed to multiply my own personal workload!

In choosing not to delegate those simple duties around the house, not only do I remain busy running around picking up clothes, taking out the trash, and washing dishes, but I'm also not giving the kids that sense of pride we all get when we pitch in and help a little bit. Most importantly, by not handing over some responsibility, I'm training the kids to be entitled jerks when they get older. God knows, we don't need any more of those. A sense of belonging can come from just participating a little.

Just for argument's sake, let's say that the only reason you agreed to have kids was so you would have some dependable help around the house. The plan was that, as you get older and weaker, these children of yours would be getting stronger and presumably taller, and as time passed, you'd be able to off-load certain domestic duties onto them so you could shuffle off to the easy chair, beer in hand.

But as with most things, your dream of couching it into the sunset years with your own staff has slowly begun to crumble. The kids did indeed get stronger and taller, but you found it a different story to actually get them to do your bidding.

Plus, they developed opinions of their own and a little attitude to boot. To make matters worse, they actually disagree with you on some things and your inner Rodney Dangerfield begins to emerge.

Don't let this happen to you!

Behold, the power of tricks and manipulation. I already explained that coming up with creative ways to get your kids to help out around the house is key. You want to make whatever it is sound so fun and challenging that they'll surely want a piece of that action regardless of what it is. If you make it sound fun they'll want to at least try it.

One sure way to get the kids engaged is by framing things as contests, or challenges where they can win prizes like time on the computer or television. Kids will do most anything if you offer something fun or delicious in return!

Don't offer any thing specific yet. Just assure them that it's something really cool and they'll want it. Then figure it out later. If you offer something specific, you run the risk that it's something they don't want, and you'll be dead in the water.

Big picture: As people with kids, sometimes we have to be less concerned with the immediate result of our instruction, and consider how our parenting will manifest down the road when it matters most.

By now we all know that when attempting to task our kids with chores around the house, it's best to show them that some jobs can be thought of as games, and that getting things done can actually be fun.

In that vein here are a few ways to hopefully get your kids to enjoy helping out. Ready, get set, go!

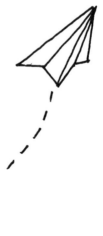

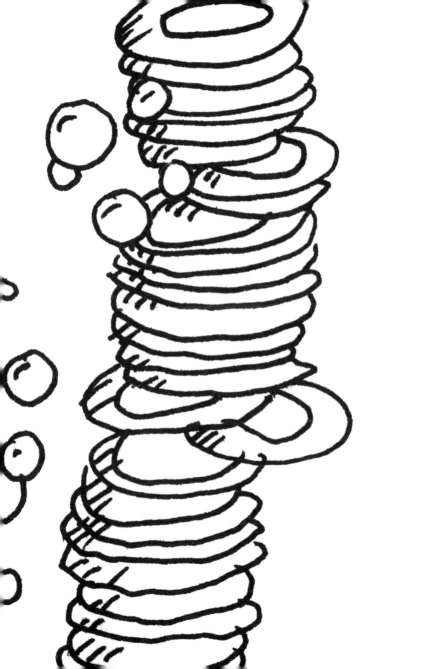

13. REDESIGN YOUR ROOM!

Keep Kids Busy For:
45–60+ minutes

You Will Need:
- *Towels*
- *Oven mitts*

Ah yes, the ol' "cleaning of the room." One of the most traditional family battles waged between parent and child.

Sometimes, we all get stuck in the house for an entire afternoon for reasons like bad weather, illness, or any number of life's little surprise travails. Spending that unplanned day at home from our regularly scheduled programming requires some quick thinking and fancy footwork.

If they're well enough, and their rooms need cleaning, here's a way to make getting that job done in a fun and possibly unexpected way!

Though you might have to redefine what you consider to be "clean" for this to work.

It begins like this. You say to your horde, "Hey guys, I have an idea! Why don't you go and arrange your room any way you want today! Be your own interior decorator! You can move your bed any way you want or hang up some new posters."

Their confused looks will indicate that those rusty gears are slowly grinding into action and a green field of possibilities is unfolding before them. It's important at this point to mention that there will be no digital access for the next couple of hours. Taking that off the table usually helps the process.

At first they might think you're trying to trick them into cleaning their room, which of course you are, but by giving them ownership of their space, you're betting they would actually want to make it clean. Even if it's their kind of clean, it's probably better than the way it is currently.

So, if this idea sparks some interest, you did it correctly and should get some questions like, "Can we put our beds in the middle of the room?"

"Sure," you say.

"Can we hang all our pictures upside down?"

"Sure," you say.

"Can we get a hamster?"

"Let's talk about that later," you say.

Just a quick note, which you probably already know: Never say "No." Always "We'll see" or "Let's talk about that later." These responses are easier to say and easier to hear. We hated it as kids and your kids will hate it too. But it works!

When it's raining out, and everyone is getting a little light on ideas, kids will show interest in the darndest things! Plus, your kids will realize that it can be great fun to re-arrange your room, moving things around, putting up new posters, all of that! If you're really going for it, you can entice them with a reward like a new poster or you will paint a square of chalkboard on one of their walls with some chalkboard paint!

I can remember being home inside for an afternoon during a snow day. I must have been twelve or thirteen. I came up with this idea on my own. I just started moving things around, taking posters down. The noise did attract the attention of my mom, and her reaction was perfect. She didn't freak out. She calmly laid down a few rules ,which I suggest you lay down as well, and left me to my work.

Rule 1. *When you're done the door has to open and shut without hitting anything.*

Rule 2. *You need to be able to walk into the room without crawling over something to put away clothes and/or vacuum.*

Rule 3. *No scratching the wood floors (which is how I*

learned that putting washclothes or oven mitts under things like the legs of my bed or under my dresser would make things easier to move while saving the floors from the huge gashes that would have resulted otherwise).

Rule 4. *You have to be done by bedtime.*

Her rules seemed perfectly fine to me. So, I shut the door and continued. I loved doing this. Being in charge of my own space was super fun and empowering. I didn't emerge until hours later.

I used pants and T-shirts under the legs of my bed and big furniture to protect the floors, and that allowed me to slide them into place easily. My mom would come to check on my progress, but we had to talk through the door, as I was unable to open it during most of the day.

By the end of the day, I had a completely new space. I set up a cozy "workstation" with freshly sharpened pencils where I would do my homework. My bed was placed against the opposite wall and made with different blankets, I arranged all my books by color, cleaned out my closet and made it another little work space/hideout.

This, like many of the activities in this book, requires parents, babysitters, and other caregivers to "let go" a little bit. You gotta give a little to get a little! That and kids generally respond favorably when offered the illusion of independence.

Anyway, if we all have to be cooped up in the house together because of the weather or because of the zombie apocalypse, we might as well get creative and see what happens.

Luckily you own this book and many of these activities are designed so we don't have to give too much! Ask anyone, what do I always say? "Low effort, high yield."

But, sometimes it doesn't work, in which case you can just re-gift this book to a friend with kids a lot smarter and cooler than yours. Or just toss it out. I already made the sale.

WARNING: *Depending on the type of kids you have, you might need to make sure they understand that their bedroom still needs to function as a bedroom when they're finished. Also, you may want to keep an eye on their progress so they don't bite off more than they can chew. They should be finished by bedtime.*

HINT: *I mentioned this before, but it bears repeating: If you have wood floors, give the kids towels and rags to put under the legs of their beds and dressers to protect your floors. This also makes the furniture easier to move. Oven mitts are fantastic for this purpose.*

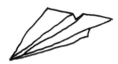

14. SOCK MATCHING SPEED TRIALS

Keep Kids Busy For:
10–20 minutes

You Will Need:
- *Clean fresh laundry*
- *Lined paper*
- *Pen*
- *Timepiece or cooking time*

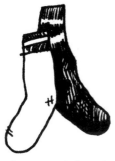

The most arduous of domestic duties, in my opinion, is laundry. More specifically, it's the folding and putting away of the laundry that really gets to me.

After many vain attempts to get the kids to help in any way, I devised a new tactic. I made a special little game of it, a competition if you will.

I turned sock matching into a game of skill and speed. Basically, I elevated the task into something one could place bets on. The game is simple. You go about sorting and folding as usual, and toss any socks you come across into a pile as you probably already do if you fold your own laundry. Once all the socks have been collected, grab a pen, some paper, and pull out a timepiece with seconds to keep time. (I use the stopwatch app on my phone for this.)

I have found that if you call the kids into the room where you've been folding, they can immediately sense they're walking into a trap. So, it's better if you bring the pile of socks into neutral territory, such as onto the living room floor or the kitchen table. For some reason simply changing location turns that confusion into curiosity!

Depending on the size of the pile, you might want to cut it down by half, so as not to shock them. Maybe start with a dozen or so socks equaling six pairs to get them started.

"Hey guys, I have a new game for us to try!" you say with uncharacteristic enthusiasm. They approach cautiously. "I'd like to see who is better at matching the socks while I time you. Everyone gets to try and the winner gets a prize."

Getting down to it is easy. We begin by tossing the socks around a little bit to build the tension, then bust out some paper and the timer.

The first contestant takes his or her place in front of the socks with hands held up. 1, 2, 3, go! Hands and socks are flying everywhere for a couple of seconds and then pairs start to appear and are set aside. The socks must be tucked into each other for them to be counted as a pair.

When the player is finished hands go up and time stops. NEXT!

I know what you're thinking. "This isn't getting you any closer to getting those socks in the drawers." True, you bring up a good point. It's not getting us any closer to being done with the laundry. But what we're doing is sowing seeds, remember?

Now, when I'm doing laundry, my kids interrupt to match socks and see if they can improve their time. Like I said, it's a long con, people—work with me here.

WARNING: *Nothing really to warn you against here, other than to make sure the laundry is completely dry. If the socks are the least bit wet, they'll never dry once they're rolled up into pairs! Duh.*

HINT: *Make it fun. Don't get angry if the kids get bored with this game after a couple rounds, leaving you with a bunch of socks still to match.*

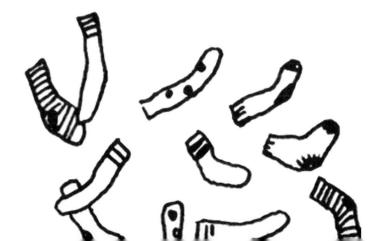

15. HOW 'BOUT CLEANING THE CAR?

Keep Kids Busy For:
45–60 minutes

You Will Need:
- *Hose water*
- *Soap*
- *Bucket*
- *Sponges*
- *Vacuum (if it gets that far)*

There is a slim minority out there who might think it cruel to order your kids to clean your car. But it's truly one of the great joys of having children, even if you have to pay them a couple of bucks to do it.

Having a car cleaned professionally costs easily $20 or $30, plus you have to pack everyone up and drive over there. Then while you're waiting for a team of strangers to do the job, dragging a dirty vacuum tube across your seats, your daughter wants you to buy her some gum. Forget it. I have a better idea.

Here's what I propose: Sit back, relax, and hand the kids a bucket and a couple of sponges and tell them that when they're ready, you'll bring out the vacuum for them.

When thinking about doing something like having your kids clean your car, it's important to hold something over their heads to ensure they will do a decent job. Since they're kids, they'll never learn the value of things unless something they value might be either given to them or taken away.

Cars are personal spaces. This country's superior idea of itself has been built on four wheels. The car is freedom, a temple, a statement. And a clean car has the ability to give us the illusion that everything in life is fine and all is in its proper place. So, would you allow a bunch of strangers with a bucket of soapy water get anywhere near your temple? Heck no.

Instruction can be easy. But first you need to take some time and get the car prepared to be violated. I suggest you begin by staging out the process.

Stage one: The exterior. This requires you to lock the car. Every parent knows that if you didn't lock the car, the interior would be as soaked as the exterior. No fledgling car wash professional needs to get inside your car for any reason. *Their first job is to clean the outside.*

Stage two: The inside. Funny thing about getting kids to clean the car, when it comes to cleaning the inside of the car, their friends mysteriously need to go home, and suddenly, they're all exhausted. It's helpful to see the glass half full. In this, if your kids' friends peter out when they catch sight of you bringing out the vacuum, so be it. You got the outside clean.

WARNING: *Make sure your kids are old enough to do this. Giving kids that are too young a job like this might attract unwanted attention from your neighbors, not to mention could result in damage to your car!*

HINT: *Don't tell your kids to fetch the cleaning supplies. This is your job and make sure they know to only use what you give them! No steel wool or hand soap!*

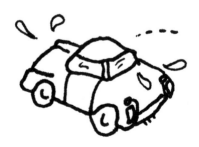

16. YE OLE WASH AND DRY

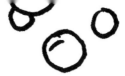

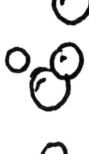

Keep Kids Busy For:
20–30 minutes

You Will Need:
- *Water*
- *Dirty drinking glasses*
- *Dirty dishes*
- *Soap*
- *Towel*

One of the easiest chores to get the kids on board with is washing the dishes. It happens every day, and it's conveniently broken into two specific duties: washing and drying. Perfect for two kids.

There are a few ways to make the chore a little more fun. One way is to allow the one who agrees to wash to pick out some music to play while they work. That might result in the one who dries wanting to switch midway, which could be a good thing. Fresh hands!

Another way to get the motivation going is to work out a grading system to how well the kids are doing. Make it simple and not based on speed!

A realistic grading system could be something like the following:

1 = A perfect score! Super clean, good job!
2 = Nah, gotta redo this one. Try again.

Now, if the washer gets to pick the music, the one who dries gets to do the grading, or you can make it a team effort and you do the grading upon completion of all the dishes!

Of course, if a perfect score is decided it will have to result in some tangible reward in addition to the warm feeling they'll get with the knowledge that they pitched in and helped out.

If the activity works, it might just encourage the kids to want to do more than just wash the dishes! If that's the case, keep the grading system going as an alternative to just shelling out an allowance. Keeping the reward performance-based is always more effective for both parties.

WARNING: *Make sure everyone knows that this is not a race! No one wins if dishes get broken or someone cuts themselves.*

HINT: *Hopefully this will become a regular thing. If it does, switch up the jobs so no one gets stuck always washing or drying.*

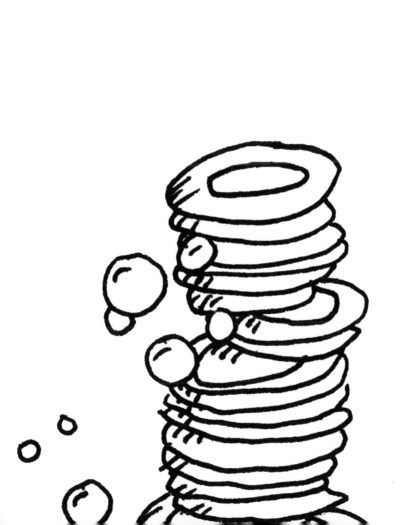

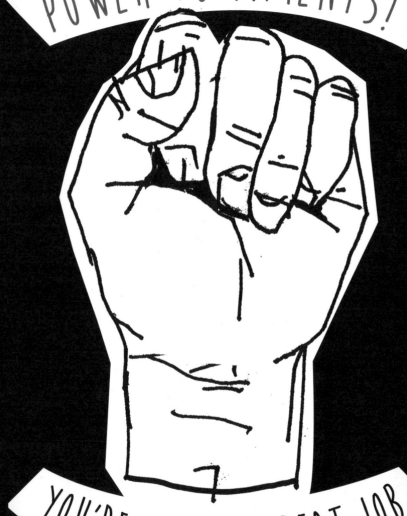

YOU DON'T NEED ME TO TELL YOU

that being a parent is a hard job. "The hardest job around!" some might say, but we persevere, and we make it up as we go along.

At least that's what my parents said when my son was born as they proudly handed me a new paperback copy of *How To Raise A Puppy*. Turns out having a puppy is a lot like having a human baby; only thing is the human baby is dumber and harder to train.

At first we settle with just hearing that our darling little miracles are out there in the world saying "please" and "thank you," at least for the first decade or so.

When people come up and say things like "Your Jonny is such a polite little boy," or "Your little Echinacea is so gentle with the little kids on the playground," we are genuinely gratified. And rightly so! Then, alas, they grow up and those kinds of precious rewards become fewer and farther between.

Still we persevere.

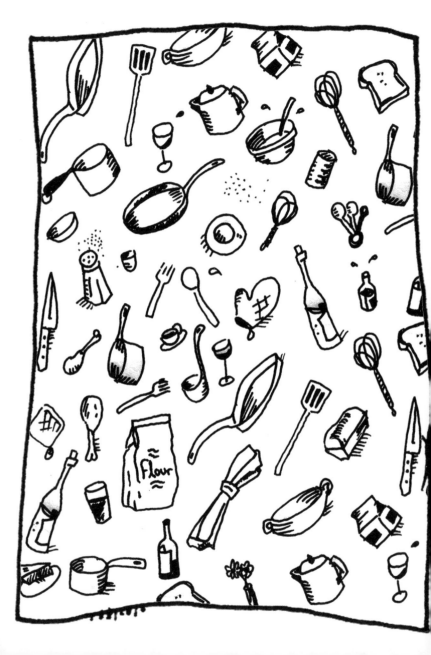

CHAPTER THREE:
GETTING KIDS IN THE KITCHEN

There's no doubt about it. Food as a *thing* has become quite trendy over the past decade. On any given day there are easily about a dozen television programs having something to do with food and cooking. Everyone and their brother has a food blog or say they do, and I can't even keep track of all the pop-up kitchens and eateries happening every weekend. Of course, I live in a foodie mecca. But still I believe many of us have a slightly adjusted attitude about what we eat and buy now versus when we were kids.

But food is also an immensely divisive topic. Being even slightly concerned about what you eat can easily put you at odds with those who will label you a "foodie" and decide you're just a stuck-up classist wanting to take their Big Macs away. Which may or may not be true. Suffice it to say that being concerned is one thing, being informed is another.

Where my kids are concerned, I try to be as informed as possible and make my decisions accordingly. Trend or no trend, it is incredibly important to be informed about what we call food, how it's grown, and why we're eating it. Besides what we eat and how we eat, it says leagues about us individually, as well as our culture.

Then there are the kids. The kitchen presents an infinite amount of teachable moments. Big life stuff really. Knowing how to shop for food, choose a ripe melon, and cook basic dishes is huge to leading a confident and healthy life.

The ultimate goal here is to demystify the whole thing for them so they can feel comfortable and empowered enough to cook and make decisions about food. We want to raise kids who don't feel that opening a box or peeling back the foil is cooking.

Of course, if you have already introduced them to cooking, great! You're ahead of the game. If you haven't introduced your kids to the wonders of the kitchen, you're in for a great time, but first you have to lighten up and stop thinking your kids will slice off a finger.

This is a great opportunity to begin a valuable tradition. This is the training that will hopefully result in your kids becoming well-adjusted adults. You want that, right? They might not become world leaders but they might be able to take over the household cooking duties every once in a while.

It might seem daunting at first, but getting your kids comfortable in the kitchen is easier than you might think. It's getting yourself comfortable that might be the real work!

Start with small projects, and eventually/hopefully you can park it at the counter with a glass of vino and bark orders, while your little ones take over.

In this next section I'll talk about some fun activities in an attempt to break down the barrier some of us have when it comes to letting the kids in the kitchen and some others that might start introducing some good conversations.

I'll set it up, then you kick the goal. You probably know this already, but remember to explain to the kids that whenever they do any project in the kitchen, they should always try to keep a clean work area and wash their hands often.

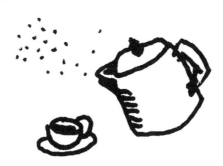

17. DINNER MENUS

Keep Kids Busy For:
30–45 minutes

You Will Need:
- *Paper*
- *Pens*
- *Markers*

The best way to get the younger kids interested in what's going on in the kitchen is by giving them a job where they get to see the big picture and what all goes into preparing a meal.

Helping to plan the dinner along with little menus for the family on a regular night is a great way to keep them occupied post-homework while giving them something fun to do that's tied into a family routine.

I used to love to play restaurant as a kid. I'd get dressed up and pretend my restaurant was a super fancy spot and required a jacket and tie. Then I'd make a seating chart with name placards. I offer this little side duty because I know some kids might not want to stop at just making menus.

As most things it's always good to lay out a few ground rules. Especially when working in or around the kitchen.

1. Never yell at the staff.

2. Always say "corner" when coming around a blind corner.

3. Always wash your hands.

4. The customer is always right.

5. Always seat happy, hip-looking people near the window.

6. There are no choices or substitutions to the menu items.

7. It's over when Mom / Dad say it's over.

Of course, you can add or subtract as needed.

Once you're all in agreement with the house rules you can begin.

If you can plan this activity ahead of time, you can actually plan out the meal together. But if there's no time for that and you're putting this activity into play at the last minute, still try and take a second to sit down with your child and tell them what you're planning. This will also get you to think a little bit about what you're doing, especially if you're like me and practice a kind of kitchen MacGyver almost every night!

You can begin by letting them know what you're planning and help them write it all down before they go off and start designing their menus.

Depending on what you're having, bread could also be included. Water or other drinks could be made available for the sake of a full-looking beverage menu. If your kid wants to have more menu choices, tell them that fixed nightly menus are what all the finest restaurants are doing now.
Once the kids get all the info written down, tell 'em to get lost and go create their masterpieces. Dinner in 15 minutes!

They will eventually start coming up with additional ideas of what they want to do. For the most part, let them do what they want, just as long as they remember the rules.

Eating with the family is not only a nice way to check in with everyone at the end of the day, but it also can be an important time for the family to just be with each other and bond for a couple of quick minutes, or however long.

I know that it's hard to get the family to sit down together every night, but this activity can help to get everyone to think about food, create something together and on their own, and be together.

WARNING: *Make sure you get the kids to sign on for clean-up duties. They might just be a little more important than set-up duties!*

HINT: *Keep the menu simple. Simple is best, so do not get overly complex. To add a little more fun to this activity, perhaps your kids would like to play waitperson too! Let them take orders and if they can handle it, maybe they can even serve! Proceed with caution.*

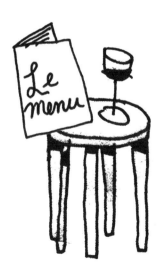

18. NAPKIN RINGS

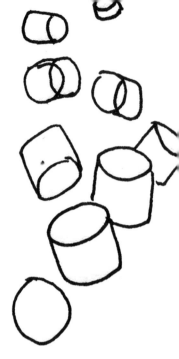

Keep Kids Busy for:
30–45 minutes

You Will Need:
- *Paper*
- *Scissors*
- *Pens, markers*
- *Glitter*
- *Craft supplies*

Really? Napkin rings? Yep. They're easy and you can use almost anything to make them. Remember this is about keeping kids and their little hands busy!

We don't really see too many of these things on the modern dinner table today—at least I haven't.

What are they used for anyway? Where do they come from? The napkin ring, also called a "serviette" ring (*serviette* is another word for napkin), was originally used to identify the napkins of a certain household or family in France, as were most things of the culinary ilk, during the 1800s. By the end of the nineteenth century napkin rings made their way across the westernized world and we began to see them on dinner tables in the United States.

Most napkin rings at the time were made of silver or bone, wood, porcelain, or glass among other things, but today you can use almost anything.

This is a fun project for fancy table settings on occasions like Thanksgiving, but why not make it a regular routine in your repertoire of kid-friendly activities?

It's easy and it beats having to fold and refold your "serviette" every night.

Since the materials could really be anything, you can make this a friendly competition. Who can make the most colorful or the most creative napkin ring? (not biggest!) Competitions are great ways to get the littles onboard and get them involved with a fun activity.

HINT: *Direct the kids toward whatever stock of materials you might have a lot of and lying around, such as extra cardboard, construction paper, old newspapers, plastic cups . . .*

WARNING: *Remember if they go for the recycling, ask them to rinse and dry anything they might want to use. Nothing sticky is allowed on the dinner table, and that goes for glue. Good luck.*

19. BLIND TASTING

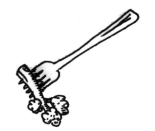

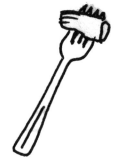

Keep Kids Busy For:
30–45 minutes

You Will Need:
- *Random food and food-like items*
- *Forks and spoon*
- *Blindfold*

We are all familiar with what a blind taste test is. Instead of choosing one of two of the same type of food or drink, make this a full-on guessing game of multiple foods!

This is a great way to put all those crazy ingredients you've collected and barely used to good use. I'm sure if you go and look in your fridge or any of your cupboards right now, most of you will find two or three items no one has touched possibly in years. Cans of beans, tubes of odd spicy pastes, or tins of oily fish might be among them. Full disclosure: That's what I found in my own kitchen not too long ago. All items were collecting dust, but still perfect for confusing young minds and taste buds.

First, let me begin by saying that your involvement here may be required a bit more than most of the activities I include in this book. Of course you know your kids better than

I do, so follow along and if you feel OK to leave them alone, do it.

As we've discussed, most kids adore a good competition or challenge. So by making this a competitive challenge, you have a good chance at getting your kids onboard. The first question they'll probably ask is if you plan on making them eat anything weird like bugs or anything moldy. Hint: Say, "No."

A fun thing about a blind taste test is that the kids have to kind of trust you. And as any parent knows, winning over your child's trust, especially as they get older, is never easy. Hehehe. . .

To begin, set up a table with a pen, a piece of paper, some spoons, and four or five small covered containers with the mystery food already in them. You want to have everything ready to go so they don't hear you rooting through the cabinets or the refrigerator. If they hear where you are in the kitchen, they'll be guessing rather than tasting. Finally, you'll need a good blindfold.

Feed each blindfolded kid a small spoonful of each of the five foods set before them.

As they taste each sample write down what they get right. Train them to identify each item by describing it as carefully and as colorfully as they can. Get them to use fun descriptions like salty like the ocean, crunchy like a desert, or leafy like a jungle. Encourage them to use their words! This way you're not only expanding their palates, but you're also helping them describe things in illustrative and creative ways. Throw in some yummy sweet things to keep them wanting more!

WARNING: *Make sure you check the expiration dates on all the items you plan on using. This is a super fun activity, but no one needs to get sick.*

HINT: *Choose a wide array of textures and flavors, and have everything at the ready before you get started. Throw in some yummy treats as a reward for playing!*

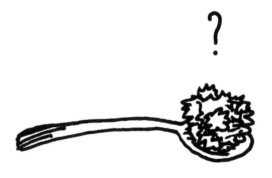

20. SMASHED-UP POTATOES

Keep Kids Busy For:
5–10 minutes

You Will Need:
- *Cut, boiled, and strained potatoes*
- *Butter*
- *Milk*
- *Salt*
- *Bowl*
- *Mashing tool*

There are some easy first-timer recipes perfect for little hands, and mashed (or smashed) potatoes is one such recipe. Besides, who doesn't love them? And when done correctly, mashed potatoes can be an incredible addition to a meal or all on their own!

To get started we need to pick the perfect potato, which means we gotta talk starch. It's the most important consideration when picking a potato to mash. It's super easy for anyone to get confused about which potato to choose as there are literally dozens of types out there to choose from.

Hands down the best potatoes to use for mashing are either russets or Yellow Fins. First, the russets. Russets might not be the sexiest potato out there, but they are high in starch, making them ideal for perfect French fries, mashed potatoes, or just wrapping in foil and baking. Yum!

If the russets are too pedestrian for you, you can go with another all-purpose potato: the Yellow Finn. They are a medium starch potato. You might be familiar with this type for their golden-yellow color and creamy texture, which make them the chef's choice for gratins or just throwing in a pan with some oil and roasting. They're also great choice for mashing.

In all honesty, making mashed potatoes is pretty easy. That's precisely why I'm suggesting it as a great way to get your kids in the kitchen and cooking.

You can easily pull up dozens of recipes for mashed potatoes on the web. This is a basic one that I use. Recite the following directions to your little one from your comfortable spot at the counter. Be there to help, but try not to hover!

Cooking the potatoes:

1. First, wash and cut 2 pounds of potatoes into small 1" cubes.

2. Fill a large pot with cool water.

3. Add a couple of dashes or pinches of salt to the water and bring to a boil.

4. Once the water comes to a boil, add the potatoes slowly without splashing and cook till tender but still firm. This should take about 15 minutes.

5. Drain the potatoes, keeping them in the pot. Things are pretty hot right now so be sure to use oven mitts and stay clear of the steam when draining.

6. Add 2 tablespoons of butter and 1 cup of milk into the steaming drained potatoes and begin mashing.

I suggest using a hand masher for kids rather than an electric beater. An electric beater is fine for kids who may have used one before, but for newbies, an electric beater might result in you cleaning fresh mash off the ceiling. Besides, doing things by hand is always the best way to start off!

Continue mashing until all the milk and butter has melted in and the potatoes are creamy! Yum!

Once your kid gets this basic mash process down then you can add ingredients like feta cheese, a little chicken broth, or a dash of Italian parsley for a smidge of color when serving.

WARNING: *Like any cooking activity with kids that requires heat, making smashed potatoes is a project that works best with an adult present.*

HINT: *The skin of a potato actually has more nutrients than the meat of the potato. Take advantage of this and keep the skins on! Just wash the potatoes well before slicing them into one-inch cubes to be added to the boiling water. Your mash will look nicer too!*

MASHER ⟶

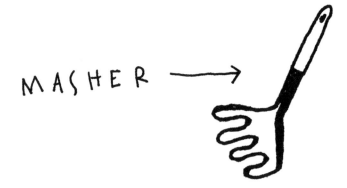

21. OVEN-POT BREAD

> **Keep Kids Busy:**
> *2 hours*
>
> **You Will Need:**
> - *Flour*
> - *Instant yeast*
> - *Salt*
> - *Water*
> - *Bowl*
> - *Plastic wrap*
> - *Parchment paper*
> - *Vegetable oil*
> - *Oven-safe pot with lid*

Quick question: What's better than sliced bread?
Answer: Freshly baked sliced bread! Duh.

As a lad, I was lucky enough to have a mom who not
only liked to bake, but was actually good at it.
For a few years during my growing up, my mom would
bake all our bread. As a result, on a regular basis we
had that incredible smell of baking bread permeating
the house on a weekly basis. To this day I can't pass a
bakery without thinking of my mom's bread just out of
the oven! Suffice it to say, there are very few things that
smell as magical as baking bread.

As a treat, just as the bread would come out of the oven, she would slice into one of those amazing warm loaves and give us all a thick slice with butter and honey.
I'm actually salivating as I write this.

Funny thing is, making bread is one of the last things most of us think to do, and one easiest things to make! Not to mention the payoff is huge and everything it's cracked up to be. It's the absolute definition of "High yield, low effort!"

Recently, I came across a recipe perfect for those of us who haven't baked in a long time or have never baked bread. It's a loaf that bakes entirely in a sturdy pot rather than loaf pans.

I gave it a try not too long ago and was pleasantly surprised at the easy assembly and the finished product. You can spread this out across two days when you include letting the dough sit, but it's worth it! It comes out light and fluffy with a good crust and it tastes pretty darn good. So good, in fact, that I decided right then and there to include it in this book. So, without further ado, preheat the oven and let's get started!

Again, like most things in this book, try and let your kids do most of the work.

Don't be surprised if the smell of your baking bread attracts a few folks into the kitchen. For that reason, I suggest doubling the recipe to make a couple of loaves at the same time. I guarantee that one of them will be gone in no time.

Sure, some kinds of bread are more difficult than others, but do yourself a favor and don't worry about that right now; pull together these few ingredients and make some gosh-dang bread already!

For this recipe you'll need:
3 cups of bread flour

1 teaspoon active of dry yeast

1 teaspoon of salt

1 ½ cups of water, warm

1. *Start off by mixing the flour, yeast, and salt in a 3–4 quart bowl, then add your water and stir until the dough is mixed well. Your dough should be sticky looking. Cover and seal the bowl with some plastic wrap and set aside someplace warm for 6–12 hours, overnight is fine.*

2. *After 6–12 hours, check your dough. It should have visibly doubled in size! Preheat your oven to 450 degrees. Place a cast iron Dutch oven or any sturdy pot with a heavy lid that's suitable for the oven into the oven while preheating for 30 minutes to get it warm and ready. Meanwhile, take the risen dough from the bowl and place it onto a floured surface. The dough will still be very sticky. Then with floured hands, gently shape the dough into a round loaf by tucking it underneath itself, making sure there's enough flour on the surface so dough doesn't stick. This is a fun part for the kids!*

3. *Carefully take the warm/hot pot from the oven and quickly wipe the inside with a little vegetable oil with a paper towel, then gently place your rounded dough into the pot. Cover with the lid and place back into the oven and bake for 30 minutes. After 30 minutes remove the lid and continue cooking for another 10–15 minutes. Gently shake the loaf onto a cooling rack and enjoy the incredible aroma. Give it a chance to cool just a tad before cutting into the loaf, but don't wait too long. You want to slice off a thick piece for you and your helpers while it's still warm. Now sit back and prepare for the hordes to arrive in the kitchen!*

WARNING: *As with most activities that take place in the kitchen, you must be somewhat present and take the skill level of your kids into consideration before pouring your glass of wine. Also, consider sitting in the kitchen rather than on the other side of the counter or over at the table. As in any project in the kitchen, make sure you keep a clean work area and wash your hands.*

HINT: *Double this recipe if you can. Also, make sure you have butter and honey close at hand when you take the loaves out of the oven. #youcanthankmelater*

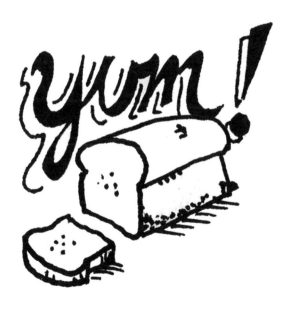

22. SETTING THE TABLE

> **Keep Kids Busy For:**
> *10–15 minutes*
>
> **You Will Need:**
> - *Forks*
> - *Knives*
> - *Spoons*
> - *Placemats*

In my family, setting the table was one of the duties my brother and I shared. Usually one of us set the table and the other cleared the table after dinner. Without fail, whoever was setting the table always asked the same questions: "Which side is the knife on?" or "Do we really need spoons?"

By most standards we were a pretty liberal family, but both my parents came from East Coast families where manners were held in high regard. Thankfully they kept up those traditional family standards to some degree.

Part of tradition were manners around the table, and a big part of that was knowing how to properly set the table.

If either of my grandmothers was over during the table-setting, the discussion of how and why salad forks were on the outside or the orientation of the knife blades would always lead to the sharing of family memories from before I was born. Tales of how strict my family was when my parents were kids were common and I loved hearing them. Sharing these stories really helps to keep important traditions alive, plus kids love to hear stories about how we parents were as kids!

So, gather the little ones around the table with piles of knives, spoons, and forks and let's do it!

Of course, I don't want to assume you don't know how to properly set a table. If you do, consider this a refresher with kids. As with many things in this book, I want to spotlight the little things we might do all the time and say, "Hold up! Let's get the kids in here!" or "Hey, why don't we make a game of this?"

There are two standard ways to set a table: informal and formal settings. The difference is mainly the amount of utensils and dishes, but both settings use a basic layout based on the more formal setting.

The arrangement of the utensils is based on how the meal unfolds and when the diner will use them. In the western world, we place the napkin, bread plate, and butter knife to the left of the plate, and the spoons, stemware, and knives to the right of the plate. In the eastern world, places such as Greece or Turkey, the opposite is true.

It's fun to sprinkle in a little "why" when learning the "how." Kids love to know why certain rules exist and how things came into existence. It helps them to construct a world with meaning around them, rather than just a bunch of flimsy facades propped up with a lot of "Cause I said so's"!

One of these questions I had as a kid was, "Who invented the fork?"

Of course there's no clear answer to that, but what we do know is that the fork replaced the knife as the primary eating utensil. It eventually found its way onto the dining table at some point during the seventeenth century and quickly became our most commonly used utensil.

The fork is also credited with kick-starting the idea of what a table setting should consist of and what other elements would accompany a meal.

Soon after the introduction of the fork, actual "rules for service" were developed, and the various levels of said service were widely adopted.

Once all these rules were developed, it was the English style of service, which we are most familiar with, that eventually became most popular here in America for its practicality versus the longer and more methodical style practiced by the French. The French style of service called for settings to accompany individual courses, each with their own fleet of specific equipment.

Of course that would have been a huge job for some unlucky kid to clean up after!

So, get the kids together and set the dang table! Don't forget to place the kids' handmade dinner menus and napkin rings. Have fun!

WARNING: *Stay close to the action during this activity. Remember you have to play the role of facilitator and storyteller here. Plus something could get broken if you wander off for too long.*

HINT: *Let the kids start off by setting the table how they think it should be. When they're done then you can show them the correct way. Maybe let them make place cards for all the guests when they're done.*

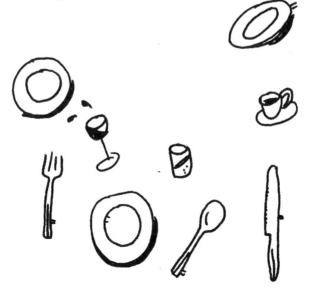

23. SHELLING BEANS

> **Keep Kids Busy for:**
> *20–30 minutes*
>
> **You Will Need:**
> * *Three bowls*
> * *Beans to be shelled*

Shelling beans is one of those kitchen chores that can transport us to a simpler time where we can slow our collective flow enough for casual conversation between friends and family.

It's easy to share the work and in no time you'll find yourselves looking for more beans to shell soon after sitting down.

With most beans, if you can get them in the shells from your local farmers market or grocer, do it. If you're lucky enough to have a garden, you might not have to go any farther than your backyard!

There are a lot of beans out there that require a little shelling. Here's a quick list of beans that are perfect for gathering the kids for a family shelling.

1. Fava beans
2. Italian butter beans
3. English peas

Whatever beans you shell, make sure you use them right away to capture the freshness and before they start to wilt.

If you happen to be working with one of my favorites, fava beans, here's an easy, kid-friendly recipe for a delicious fava puree. This is a yummy and quick way to enjoy your fresh favas on a toasted baguette! Remember fava beans have an outer shell and an inner skin. Make sure to remove both before continuing!

To begin:
Gather your helpers around a table with three bowls. One bowl for the beans to be shelled, a second bowl for the shells/pods, and the third for the shelled beans.

To make around a quarter cup of fava bean puree you'll need:

5 cups of shelled fresh favas (1½ lbs)

1 bowl of ice water, set aside

4 tablespoons of extra-virgin olive oil

Salt (just a pinch)

Freshly ground black pepper (to taste)

2 medium garlic cloves, minced

¾ cup water

Fresh lemon juice

1 sliced and toasted baguette

1. *Bring a large pot of salted water to a good and rolling boil. Add your freshly shelled favas and boil them until the bean's inside second skin turns bright green and firm but not hard, about 1 to 2 minutes. Drain your beans and immediately put them into the waiting bowl of ice water until they cool down and stop cooking. Once they're cool enough to handle, you can begin peeling the light second green skin from each bean to reveal the green inner bean and place them into another bowl and put aside.*

2. *Heat the olive oil in a medium pan over low to medium heat and add the bright green beans with a pinch of salt and pepper along with the minced garlic. Quickly stir-fry the beans and stir them while you add a little water so the beans don't dry or stick to the pan. Cook the favas and garlic for about 5 minutes or until favas are tender.*

3. *Bust out your food processor and puree the favas until smooth and transfer to a bowl. At this point you can squeeze a little fresh lemon over your puree. Serve with a sliced and toasted baguette and garnish with a little pecorino cheese, and a drizzle of olive oil if you like! Tasty.*

WARNING: *As with any project in the kitchen, make sure you keep a clean work area and wash your hands often.*

HINT: *Use an apron or have a few clean dry towels handy.*

24. EASY SALAD DRESSING

Keep Kids Busy For:
5–10 minutes

You Will Need:
- *Olive oil*
- *Vinegar*
- *Bowl or jar*
- *Fork or mini-whisk*
- *Salt*
- *Pepper*

Another super easy and fun way to introduce your kids to the kitchen is by making a simple salad dressing.

Making a simple salad dressing is one of those skills that later in life your kids can bust out at any impromptu dinner party and impress their friends! Plus, it uses typical items that you might find in any kitchen.

Of course, there are literally hundreds of salad dressing recipes out there available to anyone with web access. I always prefer vinaigrettes to the heavier, creamier dressings. I prefer to be able to taste the greens and any of the other vegetables that happen to be included, rather than a thick, pasty dressing.

Many of the recipes suggest making the dressings in a little jar to be used next time. I don't do that. I prefer to make just enough to be used every time, though I agree that using a jar with a lid for shaking the mix together is easy and smart.

The basic proportions to a very basic vinaigrette are usually 3 to 1. This means three parts oil to one part vinegar and a pinch of salt and fresh pepper to taste. As you get more comfortable and get to know this ratio, you can begin to eyeball these proportions and add your own embellishments.

First let's talk about olive oil.

Olive oil is one of those things that you should spend a little extra money on if you can.

I try to keep two kinds on hand: one more expensive kind for making dressings or drizzling on pasta. The other will be a lower grade oil for cooking. Since heat destroys much of the flavor of the oil, there's no point in using the really good stuff.

As far as vinegars, as you probably know, each has a unique flavor and many kinds can be used in this salad dressing recipe. But since you're asking, I prefer red wine vinegars or a good balsamic for dressings.

To prepare the dressing:
Have the kids grab a small bowl or a little jar and combine the ingredients. If it's a small salad, put 3 tablespoons of a good cold-pressed extra-virgin olive oil and 1 tablespoon of vinegar into the bowl or jar along with a pinch of salt and pepper.

If your kid is using a bowl, use a fork or a small whisk to combine it all.

Obviously, if you're using a jar, put the lid on and shake.

Once you get comfortable with this recipe, you can add a dollop of grainy mustard, honey, or finely minced shallots to the mix. The big thing to remember is, try not to overpower the salad with the dressing, just bring out the natural flavors of your greens.

WARNING: *Always taste what you're cooking, or assembling, in the kitchen. You can't properly season what you're making without tasting a little bit along the way.*

HINT: *Once your kids get comfortable with making this recipe, encourage them to try adding different ingredients, like raspberries!*

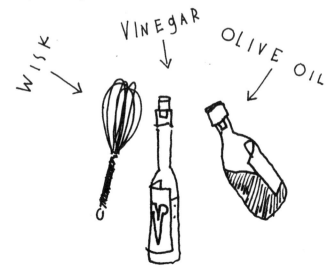

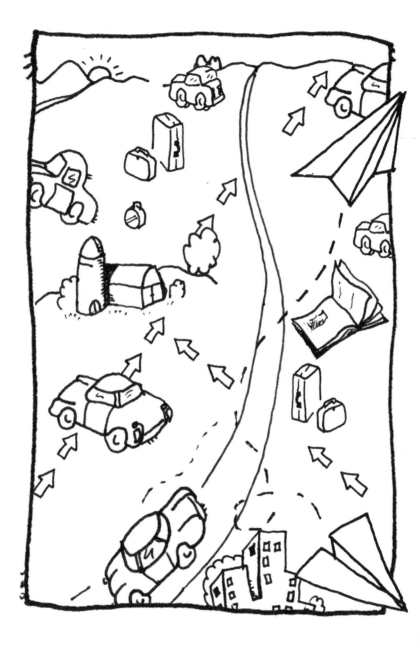

CHAPTER FOUR:
Y'ALL BE TRIPPIN'!
CAR TRIPS AND ERRANDS

As a kid I hated tagging along with my mom on endless errands or those long weekend car rides.

Then there were the road trips, ugh! Those long treks across the country would start off fun enough, but they would soon settle into a challenge for everyone.

No matter how my parents would sell them to us, car trips always meant my brother and I would be sentenced to the backseat where fresh air and unobstructed views were at a minimum, and carsickness was inevitable.

As a family, I seem to remember us driving everywhere. From Colorado we'd drive to Mexico, Pennsylvania, and even to New York. Anywhere normal people would fly, we'd drive. "See the country!" they'd say. "Family time!" they'd announce, as my brother and I fit our bodies into tight nests of pillows and blankets we'd construct in the backseat of the family Saab, preparing for the hours and days ahead.

Of course it wasn't all bad. We did see some beautiful country, travel some historic old roads, and it was great to be able to spend quality time as a family.

After a ton of hours and a ton of miles, we'd all settle into a pattern with each other and find things that would occupy us on our own, like reading, drawing, or in my case staring out the windows in effort not to get sick!

Knowing that the fun of a road trip would begin wearing off for my brother and me after roughly the first hour every morning, my parents had to do some fancy footwork to get our minds off our increasing discomfort so we could cover some ground with as little whining as possible.

It's true that the activities one can do while stuck in a car on a road trip are few and far between, and I think we can all agree there hasn't been too much innovation in this area. I'm sure I won't be offering up too many new activities here that you haven't heard of before, but I think my new variations on a few of them might make them feel like they're new. Let's see.

25. HEY KIDS, HOW MUCH AIR CAN YOU FIT IN YOUR MOUTH?

Keep Kids Busy For:
20 minutes (Could be longer. You'd be surprised.)

You Will Need:
Nothing!

One of the more popular games my father would play with my brother and me didn't have a name. A formal name didn't seem necessary.

To pull this activity out, you need timing. Knowing when it was the perfect moment to drop it on your unsuspecting victims required skill. To be clear, when I say victims I really mean kids under the age of 10.

Before I forget, for this particular activity, it also helps if your kids are tired, a bit slaphappy, and possibly bored out of their skulls.

Like I said, this game doesn't have a name, but seeing how this is a book of stuff with names, I'll call this one *"Hey Kids, How Much Air Can You Fit In Your Mouth?"* Sounds about right.

It goes like this. Picture a family of four, mid afternoon, tooling at a pretty good clip down some lonely freeway smack dab in the middle of the country. Blankets that once formed a cozy, warm nest in the chilly morning have all been kicked to the floor along with the pillows and stuffed toys.

Oh, and it's summertime. It's hot. Sweaty, middle America hot, and my brother and I are at each other's throats arguing over personal space.

This would be the point when my dad would look into the rearview mirror at us in the backseat and offer a little idea to get our minds off the heat . . . and each other.

"Let's have a contest! How much air do you think you guys could fit into your mouths?"

Of course this was a ploy to get us to shut the hell up, but it was all we needed. A good old-fashioned competition to finally decide who gets to use the middle armrest for the next hour!

On the count of three. 1-2-3 go! My brother and I would immediately begin filling our mouths with the stuffy hot car air. We'd do this gamefully for 5 or 6 minutes without any thought to what we were really doing, or the logistics of how one would actually measure the air in our mouths.

How was Dad going to tell who had the most air? Does it have to be in the immediate mouth area or could we store a little in our upper throats? Where does the mouth end and the throat begin? These were just details. Regardless of all that, we tried and tried, judged only by our dad's cajoling and sporadic glances in the rearview mirror to check on our progress while he continued driving.

My mom wasn't a fan of this particular activity.

At one point, during one of the first times we played this game, my brother and I stumbled upon an incredible innovation sure to change the game: rolling down the windows!

Now we had a rush of unlimited air forced directly where we needed it: straight into our wide open mouths! With cheeks flapping . . . now who's the winner, Dad?

Shawn and I were totally occupied gobbling up air and miming success to the other as my parents enjoyed a few minutes of relative silence and comfort knowing the kids were occupied. Meanwhile, we squirmed in silence trying to pop each other's fat, air-stuffed cheeks.

The point is that we were so ready for something, anything to do, and my dad knew it, so he used our desperation against us. A+ for parenting right there!

It's fair to say that Shawn and I would have continued longer if my mother hadn't insisted that my father stop the game. Which only upset my brother and me since we both were convinced we were each winning.

"OK, guys. Your mother says it's time up. Matt, you're pretty good at this, I think you might have won that one, but Shawn definitely was a close second!" And with that he knowingly primed the pump for the next round! Also, for my dad, this was a sly joke implying that my brother and I had big mouths.

WARNING: *Don't let your kids stick their heads or any part of their bodies outside the window. Didn't you see the 1981 Michael Caine movie* The Hand?

HINT: *Keep checking in on your kids with words of encouragement and keep the game going as long as you can. When they first try it and start giving up, tell them that was just a practice round to loosen up their cheeks, and encourage them to get ready for the real round to start in . . . 3-2-1!*

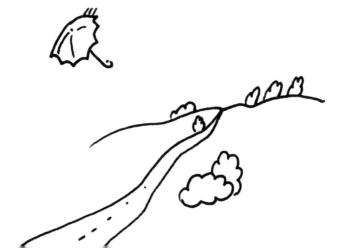

26. THE INCREDIBLE SUPER FANTASTIC HUMAN VIDEO GAME

Keep Kids Busy:
20 minutes

You Will Need:
Two willing kids in the backseat

When reading in the car makes you sick, the batteries are dead in all the kids' digital devices, Mom and/or Dad's phone are off-limits while they "charge," and inspiring ideas seem to be all tapped out, things can turn desperate. Not necessarily in a "Donner party" sort of way, more in a "mother of invention" sort of way.

This could be a magic moment when your kids start coming up with some pretty amazing ideas to keep themselves occupied on their own! All you have to do is set up the environment and they'll do the rest.

The Incredible Super Fantastic Human Video Game is one of those slightly odd ideas born out of the minds of two preteens half dead with boredom.

Let me explain. Assuming you're sitting in the backseat already, situate yourself to be sitting with your back against the inside of the car with your feet facing your backseat neighbor/sibling. The basic idea is that you—your body—is actually the video game. The game is simple. Your hands are spaceships slowly closing in on each other and the "player" uses your feet as controllers to move their ship (one of your hands) so as to not crash into the other.

The way it works is the "video game kid" sits facing the "player kid," knees up and feet resting on the heels with toes sticking straight up. The "video game" holds their hands in a "duck" form, or the shape of a spaceship pointing at each other, a couple of inches above their knees.

Now the player grabs the video game's feet like controllers and moves the ship (hands). This takes some practice and some coordination on the part of the video game, but the better you get at it, the more fun it is for both kids.

It should be mentioned that the video game has to play fair. If the player is moving the controllers, the video game has to move the ship accordingly. Things can turn ugly pretty fast if the player feels like the video game isn't being responsive and moving the ship fairly.

It can get even more fun if the video game offers lasers or torpedoes in the game. Then the player must line up the spaceship in order for it to hit whatever needs to be hit. My brother Shawn and I had something akin to the real video game Asteroids, where my brother would hold one hand up as the spaceship that could be controlled and a fist as the approaching asteroid. It was a constant battle between us.

I would complain that he was not reacting in the right way, or that the asteroid was moving too fast, and he would say he didn't feel me moving his foot.

As you could probably see, this game is full of potential problems from the user experience point of view and there really is no way to fix these very human bugs. Point is, if the situation is right, kids come up with some pretty great games! Try and remember them, log them away, then bring them up later as if you came up with them! Good luck!

WARNING: *There will be a little arguing. Lock the back doors before this activity commences and keep the seat belts buckled at all times!*

HINT: *Try and come up with a couple of quick rules before they play, like no hitting the sides of the "video game," and be easy on the controls!*

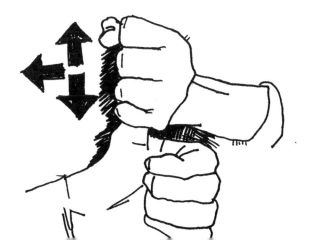

27. WHAT TIME IS IT? IT'S QUIET TIME!

> **Keep Kids Busy For:**
> *20–30 minutes*
>
> **You Will Need:**
> *Not one dang thing*

This is another one of those activities we've all done. Before I get into this one, it should be noted that some things that normally might be seen as a punishment could actually be easily rephrased into a fun and challenging competition for the amusement of all.

A perfect time to pull out this gem is when the kids are arguing or maybe getting just a little snippy with each other and you are just beginning an afternoon of errands, or a long period of time in the car.

If you are finding yourself in this position, try this: Glance into the rearview mirror with a smile and say, "Whoever can be quiet the longest gets to pick where we have lunch!" In this case you have to include a prize for the winner. It's key in differentiating this "fun" version with the punishment version.

Now put 30 minutes on the clock and quickly go over the rules.

1. *No touching. My brother and I would try to poke or pinch each other in an attempt to get the other to whimper or complain. So, no touching is a big one.*

2. *No sounds of any kind. This includes "MMMM" sounds or humming of any kind.*

3. *No pounding on the seats, clapping, or tapping the windows.*

4. *And finally, if Mom or Dad doesn't hear it, it doesn't count.*

Not surprisingly, this "game" is really difficult for kids to play. It reminds me of that challenge where you tell someone not to press the big red button, and just because you told them not to press it, it's the only thing they want to do! They want to press the big, juicy red button and that urge builds to the point they just explode. This is a truth, a behavioral flow that you can always use to great advantage in your everyday parenting, otherwise known as "reverse psychology."

Quiet Time for my brother and me was more than just a game. It was more like being asked to withstand some prolonged pain or torture without flinching. As if someone had asked us how long we could lay in a bed of snakes, or how long we could withstand having ants crawling all over us.

Prize or not, 5 to 10 minutes was usually our limit.

We'd be squirming and going crazy trying to hold all these words and sounds back from bursting out of us. But then, every once in a while, the opposite would happen. In these rare moments my brother and I would find a strange moment of peace, a calm during quiet time, and we'd suddenly be able to sit quietly for hours! Then the tides would turn against my parents. Two kids not talking would ultimately be our own sweet payback.

So, I guess as far as this one is concerned, play at your own risk. Good luck.

WARNING: *You may be unwittingly walking into a trap with this one, a trap that's easily avoided by establishing some clear rules before the game starts. Without coming right out and telling them, explain that the game must end after one hour.*

HINT: *The prize here has to be a good one. For road trippers things like controlling the radio, picking when and where you stop and get lunch, control of the middle armrest, or switching with Mom for the front seat are all quality prizes and easy to deliver on!*

SSShhhHh SSSSh

28. RE-ILLUSTRATOR, BABY'S FIRST ART BOMB

Keep Kids Busy For:
15–30 minutes

You Will Need:
- *Glossy pop culture magazines*
- *Pen*

There are those odd times when you have no option but to bring the kids along as you run around town getting the things done that can't be done online. In these desperate moments it's a good idea to have a couple of items packed for when things get difficult and you still have to stop at the store if anyone wants dinner. It's times like these that carrying some blank paper and a few pens along pay off!

Like a lot of kids, I was constantly drawing. Random doodles could always be found in the margins of my textbooks, homework, the odd phone bill, and so on. Whatever it was, if there were just a couple of inches of unused space, I filled it.

But, as things go of I wanted more. At ten years old, I was ready to move on and expand my doodling repertoire. It was right about that time when opportunity merged with inspiration. I came across a magazine while tagging along with one of my parents on an afternoon of errands. I need not remind you all that this was back in the day when kids didn't have access to any of the digital devices they have now, and keeping kids busy was a parenting skill like no other.

In most cases, it came down to whatever Mom had in her purse or could find in the glove compartment of the car. It was in the throes of a moment like this that my mom handed me a blue ballpoint pen, and while she continued to root through her bag for an envelope I could draw on, I spied a *People* magazine; or rather, a glossy opportunity beckoning from a small table next to a water cooler.

In no time, I had filled that magazine with doodles making all the fresh, happy-looking celebrities into a raunchy orgy of zombies and an assortment of black-eyed perfume models. Of course this was before the time where this kind of behavior might present a red flag to any observant parent or teacher. Boys will be boys. But most importantly, I was occupied and my mom could sit and wait in relative peace.

Of course, my mom had to discard the evidence for fear they might charge us for the missing magazine or worse yet, see the proof she had a little monster in her care. But the damage was done. I was hooked. I started drawing and transforming every magazine I could find. It was great fun, but the best part was leaving it behind! Just a little art bomb left behind by a ten-year-old budding artist becoming familiar with subverting society through expression. It was like having a prebound art book!

To do this with kids, there's not much to prepare or stock up for. You just need to keep a handful of pens (Sharpies work best) in your bag or purse.

As for the magazines, just keep an eye out for them when you're in the waiting room of a doctor's office or at an airport. Maybe it's a *Fisherman's Monthly* or, even better, a *People* or *Us* magazine. Now you can let your kids go crazy. Give them permission to craft that innocent magazine into a journal chronicling the goings-on of famous and active zombies and the bloodied, black-eyed clowns who love them!

When the waiting is over, or the doctor calls you in, place the magazine back into the stack where you found it. Leave it there for other people to "enjoy." Your job is done. Consider that waiting room #artbombed!

WARNING: *Don't get profane. Anatomical illustration is so "gas station bathroom." Remind your child that he or she is an artist. Get a little more highbrow. Zombies and long forked tongues are always preferable!*

HINT: *Don't let your kids have all the fun. This is a great activity for you too! Do some "art bombing" of your own. It's cheap and harmless, so why the heck not? Also, you can carry glossy magazines with you, but it's always more fun to come* *across random magazines wherever you find yourself waiting.*

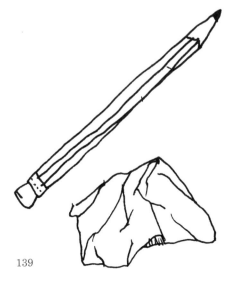

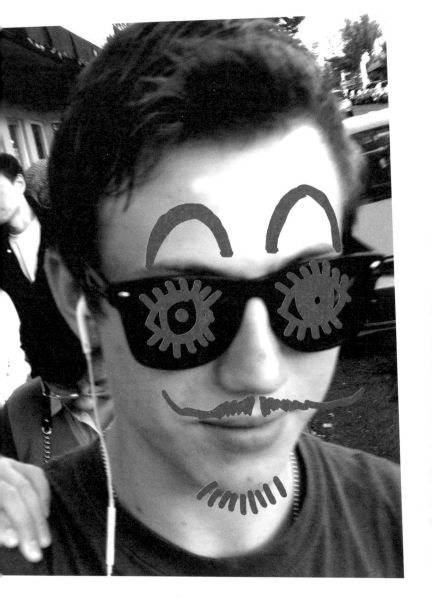

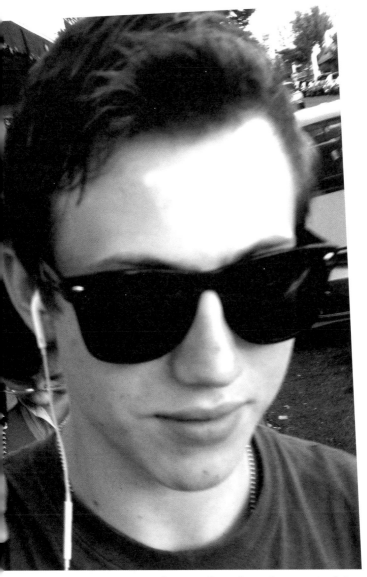

NOW YOU TRY! ART BOMB JASPER!

29. ROCK-PAPER-SCISSORS

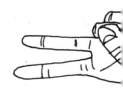

Keep Kids Busy:
20 minutes

You Will Need:
Bare hands

Another activity from the "We all have done this before" file is: Rock-Paper-Scissors. Also referred to as Roshambo, Paper-Scissors-Stone, or even ick-ack-ock, but I don't think I've ever heard anyone refer to this game as that!

Basically, I wanted to add this activity not only because it's a natural game to play when stuck in a car for hours on end, but also because after a little research, I learned of its long and rather interesting history—a story worthy of a book on its own. So look for that. Not.

First, R-P-S is a simple hand game played by two people. The game is usually played to decide something or to choose between two things. Much like rolling dice or flipping a coin.

Each player simultaneously throws out one of three possible hand gestures with one outstretched hand. Players usually count aloud 1-2-3, or "Ro/Sham/Bo!" Then on 3, or "Bo," each player forms a hands into one of the three gestures. The gestures being: Scissors, represented by two fingers extended, Rock, represented by a fist, or Paper, represented by an open hand like a sheet of paper.

The objective of the game is to select a gesture that defeats the other player's gesture. If both players throw out the same hand gesture, it's a tie. Most games end up being decided by best of three rounds. Here's how the gestures play out:

1. Rock smashes Scissors.

2. Paper covers Rock.

3. Scissors cut Paper.

The interesting history of R-P-S can be traced all the way back to ancient China. The first known actual mention of the game was in a book called Wuzazu, written by the Chinese writer Xie Zhaozhi in the Ming Dynasty, published in the 1600s. In that book Zhaozhi wrote that the game was called shoushiling, or "Hand Command," and that it actually dated back to the time of the Han Dynasty (206 BC–220 AD)!

From there the game can be traced to becoming a "thing" in Europe in the 1920s and finally landing in the States in the early 1930s. Not too sure what happened in the few hundred years between the 1600s and the twentieth century, but I'm guessing you'll survive for the time being without that additional information.

My brother Shawn and I would play this whenever we needed to decide something or if there was a question of the outcome of some other strange little game we were playing. We had no idea that there was actually a strategy or tactical approach to the game. We just thought it was a random game of chance, which of course it is on the surface, but it turns out there's tons of algorisms and strategies people have figured out about the game.

In a nutshell, this game's strategy is based on exploiting the weaknesses of your "non-random" opponents. Which means that the observant player can quickly learn the behavior of the other player, making it possible to anticipate the gesture before it's thrown into play. Another strategic tactic that has been employed by the more serious players is to shout the name of one gesture before throwing a different one—if successful, this will misdirect and confuse the opponent. I've tried this one, and not only does it confuse the other player, it really ticks them off! Good luck.

WARNING: *Before you start playing, make sure everyone agrees on the number of rounds to be played. If you don't agree from the start, this thing could go on for hours!*

HINT: *Do a little research online about various strategies out there. You might be surprised how nuanced this simple game can be.*

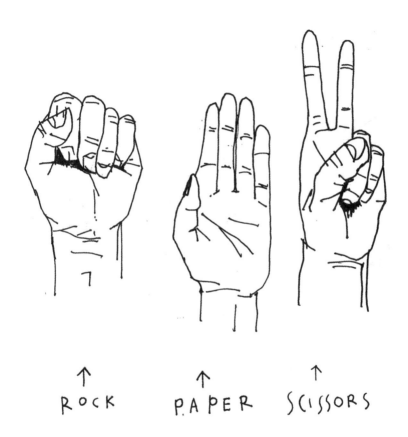

ROCK   PAPER   SCISSORS

30. MEMORY ALPHABET STYLE

In most cases, time on the road is split between silence and conversation. In most cases, the silence is split between sleeping and just staring out the window at nothing in particular. It's that part that I've grown to like more than anything else about road trippin'. Even little kids seem to appreciate a little silence in the car when driving hours upon hours upon hours.

Of the 50 percent of time spent in conversation, I would say 50 percent of that is spent playing inane little games, some of which I already presented.

For this version, we use things that we see along the road. Starting with things that begin with letter A, then B, and so on. The first person says the first thing they notice going by outside that begins with the letter "A." The next person takes the letter B and repeats what was offered for the letter "A." The next person says the first thing they see going by that begins with the letter "C" and also recalls every object that came before. So essentially you say the thing that begins with your letter, then repeat all the things that came before. The first person to stumble and forget an object loses.

It plays out something like this:

I see "A" for antelope.

I see "B" for billboard, you saw an antelope.

I see "C" for cloud, you saw a billboard, you saw an antelope.

I see "D" for Datsun, you saw a cloud, you saw a billboard, you saw an antelope.

And so on through the alphabet.

It helps to find a rhythm and clap hands in time. This makes each person want to keep the beat with their responses and makes the game a little bit more difficult. It's actually a pretty hard game. In fact, I don't think I've ever played it with someone who was able to remember the entire alphabet.

WARNING: *Continued play may result in learning the alphabet backwards!*

HINT: *For younger players that may be playing for the first time, let them take notes for the first couple times.*

31. WHAT'S THEIR DEAL?

As a child, perhaps the best part of road trips in my opinion was when we'd turn off the highway in search of a hotel or place to eat. We'd enter some little town, driving downtown along the main business route. I loved seeing that little slice of life, the local townsfolk going on with their lives in a scene totally unfamiliar to me.

Watching the townspeople doing what they do, I'd construct their life stories in my head. Names, ages, professions, all by just what I could observe, like the condition of their cars in the driveways or how they were dressed as they walked down the street.

Later, when I had kids, and they could hold conversations, I liked to point at some unsuspecting person on the street and say, "Hey, what's their deal?" In most cases, my question was answered by, "I dunno. Whaddya mean, Dad?" prompting me to provide the kind of response I wanted.

The response I was looking for, and eventually got after repeated attempts, was a made-up story based on what we could observe. I'd ask what their name could be. What are they doing? Going to work? Are they on their way to rob a bank?

With my son Jasper, our morning drives to school would be a perfect time to play this funny little people game. In fact, one of our favorite people to talk about was a crossing guard oddly stationed in front of a local grocery store, with nary a school in sight. Every morning he provided at least 10 minutes of quality guesswork. This guy was perfect fodder because of his mysterious crossing guard gig at this particular cross section, but also because this poor guy had a scrunched face that made him look really ticked off every time we passed. This detail always played an important part in our character sketches of him that built up over the year. "Hey Jasper, what's that guy's deal? Why is he so ticked off?" I'd ask. We'd laugh. Obviously he was in a rage since no kids wanted to cross his street, or because he was positioned miles from any school!

Have fun with this one!

WARNING: *Try to not let the conversation get disrespectful. Steer the character sketches towards the fantastical if you find the stories getting drab and uninspired.*

HINT: *This is a great way to start up conversations with your kids in the morning while driving them to school. Also try to encourage the kids to use different voices when describing their characters. This is also a good teaching moment to let your kids know that you can't always judge a book by its cover. Each person has a story, sometimes more interesting or bizarre than one we could ever come up with, but it's fun to try!*

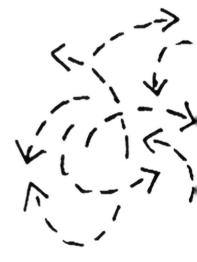

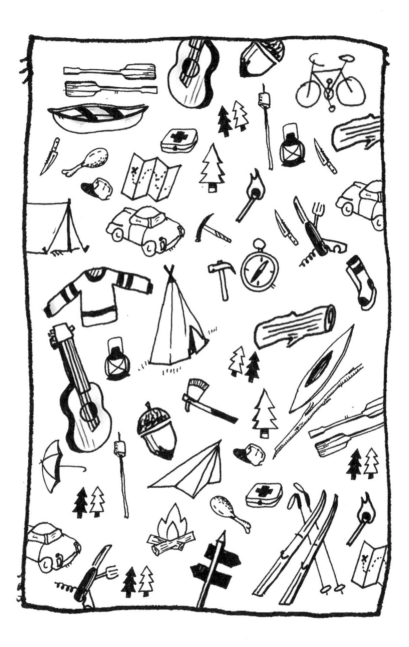

CHAPTER FIVE:
THINGS TO DO OUTSIDE

Contrary to popular belief, some kids need more than just a beautiful sunny afternoon to get their butts outside. I know . . . sounds crazy, but it's a well-documented fact that a large portion of today's youth would rather watch television or play video games than ride their bikes! Duh.

It takes a special kind of parent to pry their kids off the Internet and throw them out into a warm, beautiful afternoon, or to shove them into the car for an afternoon hike or even a camping trip. It's a hard job, but there are a couple of things you could try.

32. FOUND AROUND RAINBOWS

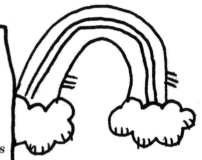

Keep Kids Busy For:
45–60 minutes

You Will Need:
- *Leaves*
- *Sticks*
- *Flowers*
- *Any other found objects*

I call this activity "Found Around Rainbows." It's fun and perfect for the backyard or camp site. It's requires a little thinking, which is nice, but kids don't seem to mind once they get started.

I really love to see what the kids come up with.
The basic idea of Found Around Rainbows is having kids create a color-coded rainbow out of items they find around the yard or some specified area, like a campground.

Start off by asking your kids to go out and start collecting colored objects such as leaves, flowers, toys, or even trash. Once the items are collected, have them place their stuff on the ground in a pattern that moves through each of the seven colors of the rainbow in order, creating a beautiful rainbow for found and natural objects. Items should represent the seven colors of the rainbow: **red**, **orange**, **yellow**, **green**, **blue**, **indigo**, and finally **violet**, or at least something close to those colors.

While it's perfectly fine to collect leaves, flowers, bits of discarded paper, etc., keep an eye on the size, and ultimately the final composition of all the items.

You don't want to collect a bunch of leaves, then have a wagon or tricycle alongside them representing red. Try to keep the size of everything within reason of each other. A little consistency goes a long way here.

Good luck and remember to take pictures!

WARNING: *Work as a group on this one. There might not be enough stuff around for more than one rainbow! Working individually on competing rainbows could result in some arguments and hurt feelings.*

HINT: *When working in a group, start some kids off by having them run in all directions, picking up anything colorful and bringing back what they find to a central location. Have the other kids stay behind and go through the collected materials and begin arranging the rainbow.*

33. POP-UP ART STAND

> **Keep Kids Busy For:**
> *A few hours*
>
> **You Will Need:**
> * *Table*
> * *Moneybox with change*
> * *Original art (cards, pictures, T-shirts)*
> * *Sign*

One of the signature summertime childhood experiences is the lemonade stand. For kids, a lemonade stand is not only about getting out there and selling your wares and making some money, but it's also about seeing how your ideas and efforts can exist out in the world. Even if "out in the world" is on the stoop right in front of your house! I like to think of the lemonade stand as your child's very first Pop-Up!

I can still recall the lemonade stands my friends and I would have. Our rickety old ironing board with a sheet thrown over it, a quickly scrawled sign that read . . . wait for it . . . "Lemonade!"

We got a stack of little two-ounce paper cups, filled a cooler with yellow, lemony sugar water, and BAM, we were in business. Alright, we weren't the players we thought we were, but a couple of bucks meant an afternoon well-spent.

Having that little stand out in front of your house is such a perfect teaching moment. A true analogy for much of what life had in store in the not-so-distant future.

This fun activity is based on all that tried-and-true lemonade stand concept except instead of selling lemonade, the kids are selling their own art.

If you had the kids do the printing activity (At-Home Printing, p. 32), this could be a perfect activity to follow that. Ideally, you would have made a slew of little cards and designs on paper and maybe a couple of T-shirts, which is the perfect kind of merchandise to sell at a little stand like this. Keep the lemonade behind the counter for folks who buy something! "Free lemonade with each purchase!" See what I did there? Marketing.

If your kid doesn't like to draw, you can swap out art and sell something your kids do like to make, like cookies or napkin rings.

To get your stand ready, begin as you would any lemonade stand set-up. By that, I mean grab some stuff to make a small counter where you can lay out your wares, create a sign, grab a couple of chairs, and locate yourself in a good spot in front of the house where you can see the kids and where they will be seen by a few passersby.

Like a lot of successful activities, this is made up of a bunch of little activities that will keep little hands busy almost all day. There's the building of the stand, the making of the sign, and the production and procurement of the artwork. Of course, you'll have to look in on the little darlings now and again, but they will be occupied, and that's the name of the game.

The Stand: *In my experience an old ironing board is perfect to keep your products up off the ground and let potential customers approach your stand at a decent height. (Old people don't like to bend over.) You could also lay a board across a couple of milk crates if you're into that hippy yard sale vibe. There's a fine line between a sucessful art stand and a garage sale. Yard sales and garage sales are not as cute as a couple of kids selling their handmade artwork, and* cute *is the operative word here. You want to market that! People always have spare change for cute!*

The Sign: *Cute, colorful signs are a surefire way to keep this from looking like some desperate junk sale. Make them big, and while you're at it, make some posters to hang through-out the neighborhood. If you do decide to make some posters to hang around the 'hood, keep them handmade; try not to make copies.*

The Product: *Have the kids go through all their artwork and pick 10 or 20 pieces to sell. As you are picking things to sell, think about price. Try for the $.50 to $2.00 price range, and since you are asking for money, try to clean the artwork* *up a little bit. Don't forget to sign and date everything! Have the kids think of titles for their work too! They might also like to hear about what the kids were thinking when they made their pictures.*

Last but definitely not least, remember: if you see the kids raking it in out there and attracting a good amount of business, fight the urge to horn in and try to sell your own crap. Pick another weekend to sell your used junk.

Looking back at my own lemonade experience, I see now where I went wrong. I needed to forget about selling lemonade and sell art! Like any budding entrepreneur about to launch his first business venture, I needed to listen to my heart! Besides, you don't need to wait for a sunny day when you're selling art. Good luck!

WARNING: *Don't let the kids enjoy the day without you! Bring your computer or magazine outside and hang out with them. Don't forget your own chilled adult beverage.*

HINT: *Get friends. This is one of those activities that might be more fun if your kid has a like-minded friend come over, share the duties, and split the profits. Business can be a lonely endeavor, and their first experience should be a fun one. There are enough little jobs in this activity for a gaggle of kids.*

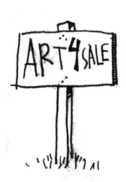

34. LET'S DO IT ON THE SIDEWALK!

You know the Beatles song "Why Don't We Do It in the Road"? The White Album? Really? Go get it.
And while you're out, grab some colored chalk.

This is an easy one. Low-hanging fruit, some might say. Chalk. It's super cheap, comes in every color you could think of, it's safe, it's not permanent, and it's something kids of all ages love to do. If that doesn't convince you then you either have some chalk already or you don't love your kids.

A single stick of chalk is a world of possibilities. Activities galore! Draw starting lines and finishing lines for races, draw a hopscotch game, random arrows and hearts to decorate your sidewalk and street, and of course scads of other ideas will come to your kids' brains.

Just hand them the chalk, kick them out of the house, and tell them to stay close to the house. Done.

Go out in about 30 minutes to check on their progress and see what masterpieces they've constructed.

WARNING: *Be sure to keep a hose handy for washing off little hands and feet before they are allowed back in the house. The hose is also handy for washing off the sidewalk if you need to for any reason.*

HINT: *The more colorful your chalk selection, the better your front walk will look!*

35. BIKE CLINIC

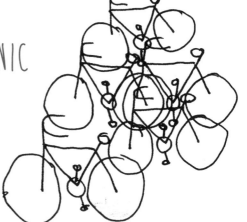

Keep Kids Busy:
45 minutes

You Will Need:
- *Your own bike*
- *Wrench*
- *Rag*
- *Lubricant oil*

Of course it depends on their age, but letting your kids take things apart and try to put them back together is a great way to learn about how things work. Or it could possibly be a great lesson in appreciating the skill of other people who know how to put things back together so they work!

I love to ride bikes. Back in the day when I was just a kid, it was freedom! I'd tool around the neighborhood with five or six of my friends. Feeling the freest a kid that age could feel.

Cruising down the middle of the quiet streets with all your friends. The wind in your hair, wranglers rolled up to your knees. We were a gang up to no good, roaming the 'hood with no agenda in mind other than to just ride our bikes.

It was like that all summer. Patrolling a six-block radius, stopping at our various houses to drink out of the hose and grab any available snacks. Some of our stops would result in a little impromptu bike maintenance.

These little clinics were spontaneous, happening in most cases while waiting on other members of our crew to show up or while we were riding and someone would yell, "Hey guys! Wait up. I gotta do something to my bike!"

Maybe a pant leg got caught in the chain, the chain fell off, or someone's tire needed air—which would require a detour to the gas station for air. Whatever it was, in most cases we'd all pull over en masse onto someone's yard and flip our bikes upside down and start screwing around with the workings.

A pair of pliers would magically appear and in minutes we'd all have our bikes in pieces. Of course, the person who needed to pull over initially just had to tighten his seat or something and he was done in the first couple of minutes after pulling over. But it was too late; we were now all neck deep in swapping seats and taking off our handlebar grips, not ready to start up again just yet.

We'd take wheels off, adjust seats and handlebars into ridiculous positions, clean pedals, over-oil chains, hose them off, and maybe add a little decoration. Basically it was just busy work that would make us all feel like we knew what we were doing. It was kind of the equivalent to popping the hood on your car and just touching and looking at stuff. Our way of feeling like big kids I guess.

Inevitably we'd try a little experimentation too. Some of us, needless to say, ended with injuries, luckily nothing too bad. Then there were other things that were cool enough for everyone to try, such as:

1. *Playing Cards: Sticking things like library cards in the spokes to make our bikes sound like they had some kind of engine installed. My friends and I would roam around together sounding like a massive swarm of angry bees.*

2. *Wipe Wash: No soap required. Just grab a hose and a rag and wipe that bike down. Remember not to wipe the chain too much. The chain needs to stay oiled so it works properly and to keep it from rusting. If you do wash and wipe the chain too much you might need to oil it up a little bit when you're done.*

3. *Handlebar Tassels: Feathers, Mardi Gras beads, Mom's old necklaces.*

4. *Extras: Reflectors, lights. Every bike should have them. And having a few extra ones never hurt anyone and can be fun to put on!*

5. *Oil: As a kid I was always over-oiling my chain and around the wheels. It's easy to do, try not to overdo it if you can. The parts on most bikes that need oil are: the chain, the derailleur assemblies, and the pedals and crank.*

WARNING: *Tell the kids never to touch the brakes on their bikes and always tighten the screws. Never use a broom handle as a handlebar! Wear a helmet!*

HINT: *This kind of activity is best if your kid's bike is a simple straight-up bike with coaster brakes and no gears.*

36. OBSTACLE COURSE

Run, jump, bob and weave = working up an appetite! When left to their own devices, kids will eventually find something to do. One of my parents' questionable parenting techniques that I have come to see as part cruel and part genius was after my mom would successfully get my brother and me outside, she would sometimes lock the door behind us. That way we couldn't get back inside and she could resume doing whatever it was she was doing. We'd see her, through the kitchen window, washing the dishes and pretending not to hear our yelling to be let back in. She knew that at some point we'd stop attracting the attention of the immediate neighbors, calm down, and figure something out. Pretty tricky and she was right . . . most of the time.

In most cases, after being tricked into going outside, we'd collected a few other members of our crew and organized a game.

In these cases I was always keen on building obstacle courses and timing each other.

The obstacle course has always been a super fun activity that most kids will jump at the chance to create.

It's got to have at least seven or eight different obstacles to be considered a real course. It has to take place just in the yard, around the house; they are not allowed to use the pets as part of it, and nothing can get broken including bones. When suggesting this activity, it helps if you mention that after they finish building it, you'll come out to time them! That always gets them!

Again, making something a competition is very effective when trying to get your kids onboard.

Make sure the kids aren't dragging stuff out of the house or the garage to be used for the course without getting permission! Otherwise it'll look like you hired a bunch of monkeys to set up an impromptu yard sale.

WARNING: *Do not attempt this activity indoors. Nothing good will come of it.*

HINT: *This is also a fun suggestion for your little animals while on a family hike. Just make sure it's in a safe area and they're allowed to go off the trail!*

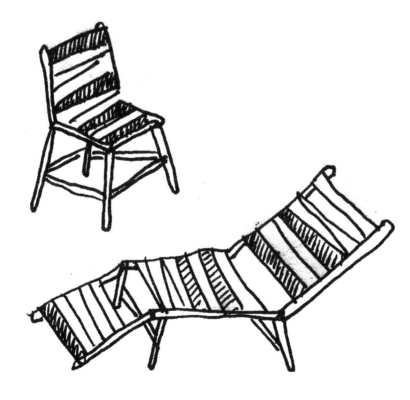

37. THOSE HOOPS BE ROLLIN'

```
Keep Kids Busy For:
60–120 minutes

You Will Need:
•   Bike wheel/hula hoop
•   Short stick
```

A true oldie and a goodie. An old bicycle wheel/rim and a short stick is all you need for hours of fun.

For today's kids, being "innovative" might mean something to do with hacking a phone or a new feature for their favorite piece of technology. But back in the day, innovation was a key to surviving long days without any sort of technical gadget! Could you imagine? No phones or video games! It's a wonder we made it through those dark days of our history!

Thankfully, through their desperation we got a lot of great games and activities. Games like Hoops and Sticks, Hopscotch, Capture the Flag, and many others. As someone said, "Necessity is the mother of invention!"

One of my favorite games that comes from this period is the aforementioned Hoop and Stick game.

It's a game of balance and momentum involving a hoop and a stick! It's pretty simple, and yet can be very challenging at the same time.

As you may have guessed, the hoop rolls along, and the stick is used to keep the hoop upright and to continue rolling.

Let's talk about what you need. First the hoop. Originally, back in the day, kids would use the metal rings from barrels, which of course you can use too if you've got an old barrel lying around. If not, I've found a metal bike wheel of any size to work perfectly fine.

For the stick, you can use really anything about 12"–14" long, such as an old drumstick, or 10" off a broom handle would work nicely too.

Once you get the rolling part down, you can add obstacles such as cones to go through, or even little ramps!

Obviously, the smaller the wheel, or hoop, the more difficult it will be. Hoops and Sticks can easily get more difficult as you play and add your own rules.

I'm aware that hoop rolling at first might not sound like something your kids will find interesting, but you might be surprised. Tell them they have to try it and help them to set up a couple of obstacles and see what happens.

Who knows, maybe they'll set up a hoops and stick neighborhood league!

WARNING: *Make sure you have a good amount of room to roll. When hoopers are concentrating on their hoops they can't be expected to look around for traffic or people at the same time.*

HINT: *Try collecting hoops of different sizes for the kids to try. Each size requires a different technique! Don't let the kids have all the fun here. Hoopin' is fun for adults too!*

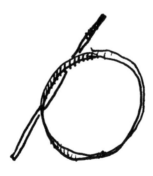

38. SAVE THE WORMS!

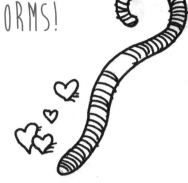

Keep Kids Busy For:
30–45 minutes

You Will Need:
A bucket

The big misconception about worms is that they come up out of their holes during big rainstorms because they're escaping their waterlogged homes. But actually, worms love the rain. Without moisture, worms would dry up and die. In addition to the rain's moisturizing powers, the rain helps worms to move faster through the wet soil. So why do they come up to the surface if it's all hunky-dory in their wet holes?

The reason they come up and onto the sidewalks is because they can more easily find potential mates on the flat surface than in their burrows. They're taking advantage of the moist earth to move up and out to find that "special" worm friend. What you see on the surface is not a mass exodus, but rather a wormy speed-dating event, and all that rain has helped by making it easier to move around.

If you happen to be holed up inside the house on a rainy day, I'm willing to bet a shiny new dime that by about 3 o'clock in the afternoon, things will be getting a little desperate and you might be reaching the end of your rope with your li'l darlings as they become desperate for something new to do.

If it has been a wet day it could be a perfect time to collect worms! Yep. That's right, squiggly little worms are great for flowerbeds and gardens, and there's never a better time to collect a mess o' worms than on a wet rainy afternoon!

So I say, Dress 'em up and kick 'em out! But before you shut the door behind them, hand them a coffee can or a plastic bucket and tell them to look in the gutters and sidewalks for worms visiting the surface, before they get smooshed by other people or cars!

This might strike a chord with the more sensitive children, which will make it a mission of mercy. Even better.

You might want to even take this opportunity to let your little team know why the little critters are showing up on the surface in the first place and how helpful they will be for the gardens!

So, send those kids out to break up the wet, wormy courtship ritual happening right outside, and tell them that they can not come back until they've "nabbed" 20 fatties for relocation. When they do get back cold, wet, and hungry you take the spoils of their adventure and toss the worms in the garden. Done and done.

WARNING: *Last but not least, make sure they wash their hands . . . with soap! Those little guys are slimy.*

HINT: *Let the kids put them in the garden, if they're up for it. Maybe give each of the worms names, too!*

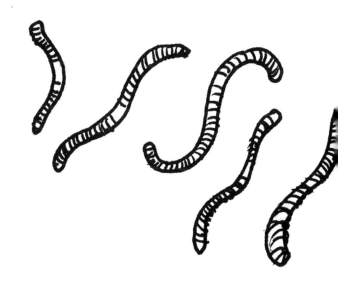

39. SHHH. THEY CAN SMELL YOU!

Keep Kids Busy For:
1–2 hours

You Will Need:
No items required

Like most parents with young children and a love of the out-of-doors, my parents had abandoned any hope of enjoying any wildlife in their natural habitat, at least while my brother and I were young. Any chance of happening across a lovely scene of a baby deer and her mother sharing a moment in a grassy clearing would be dashed thanks to our excited and loud caterwauling voices.

I don't actually remember the breaking point, but I remember a sea change in the kind of activities my father would come up with. The usual activities to engage us kids would play into our desire to be loud and crazy. I'm assuming that he felt it better to just go with it and let us enjoy the hike being as crazy and loud as we wanted.

But something happened. After years of not caring about the prospects of seeing any wildlife during our hikes, suddenly activities he would start us on seemed to be geared to keeping us quiet and a tad more respectful.

It started innocently enough. At one point along the trail my dad would stop and stare off into the distance. Standing still like a statue with a hand outstretched in our direction signaling us that we should be quiet and listen. He'd then turn slowly and say, "Did you guys hear that? I think they're watching us."

Shawn and I would look at each other then around us, slightly in fear but mostly in excitement. Were we actually going to see some wildlife on this hike?
My dad would continue, "I think I heard Them." We have to be quiet if we want to see any."

He wouldn't elaborate just exactly who or what "they" were, but Shawn and I bought it hook, line, and sinker. For the rest of the hike we were careful to keep our eyes peeled, crouching close to the ground whenever a breeze would pass, so as to hide our scent, since our dad informed us, "They can smell us and it frightens them! If we're really careful, we might actually get to see them!" He would look at us with his eyes wide and we would begin our stream of questions in excited whispers. "What do they look like? Are they dangerous? Are they big?" All these questions would be shushed with a wave of his hand as we proceeded down the trail.

"They aren't anything to worry about. They are more afraid of us." He would eventually explain.

And BANG, a simple day hike would morph into an adventurous game of hide and seek, where we were the seekers and the mysterious "They" were the "seeked."

After an afternoon of seeking we determined that "they" were not too keen on being found. My father's objective had been realized. He was able to flip the script and changed what was looking like another exercise in frustration into a relatively pleasant family afternoon in the mountains.

He didn't pull that activity out all the time, but my brother and I did use it for our own games more than a few times and at home with our friends. And I have used it with my own kids. It works like a charm. When things are getting a bit out of hand, I'd stop and say in a whisper, "Shhh. Did you hear that?"

Thinking back about that and the other odd little games my parents would throw into the situation, I realized years later, they weren't intended to be repeated every time they needed some peace and quiet. They were one-time kinda things. A way to divert our attention just long enough to get what needed to be done or fulfill an objective for the moment. Sure they can be repeated if need be, but that's not the intention. Just long enough. That's really all that is needed.

WARNING: *This game can ride along the edge of being really fun for your kids or being really scary. Know when to back off on your acting. You might never get your kids to go on a hike with you ever again!*

HINT: *Try this game any time you need a second of quiet, at home, on trips. Heck use it at work with your coworkers. A surefire hit every time!*

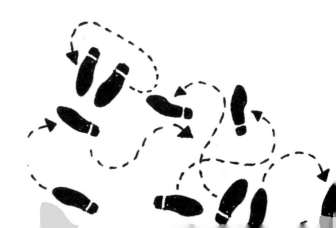

40. NATURE NAMES

Keep Kids Busy For:
1–2 hours

You Will Need:
Nada

Most every culture throughout history has employed some sort of naming tradition when welcoming its newest members into the tribe.

Names could be derived from things they saw in the world around them, such as the weather at the time of the birth, a successful harvest, or the growth of an important tree. On the flip side, it could also be as simple as passing down names held by previous generations. Some traditions would involve waiting and naming their children after certain deeds, predilections, or behaviors are observed in the child's first weeks.

Most every weekend you would find my family heading into the nearby hills for a hike and an attempted weekly communion with nature. Thanks to my brother and me, this communion could prove to be difficult. And it often became necessary for my parents to try drastic measures, which meant creatively manipulating the situation to create a desired outcome. This activity is one of the more successful ones.

It started off innocently enough on one hike when us kids were particularly ornery. Our father randomly gave us each a "Nature Name" that had something to do with our behavior at the moment. I was dubbed Thunder Foot because I was constantly running up and down the trail ahead of the family, loudly thumping, creating dust and kicking rocks. My brother was given the name Yelling Squirrel after his apparent inability to keep his voice at a decent volume and constant search of little echoes along the trail, ensuring that we never happened upon the slightest hint of wildlife, bird or otherwise.

The name was one thing we could have easily dealt with—the hard part was that my parents would only refer to us using that name for the duration of the hike. Of course, my dad named himself something like Chief Strong As Bull and my mother was Moon Princess, of course . . . ugh.

It went without saying, my brother and I would want cooler, more heroic monikers like Super Flash or Eagle Eyes, or something of that ilk.

My dad expected this would be the case. So, he would explain, that yes we could change our names, but he would

come up with them and we would have to earn them.
Wait. What? Earn them? Begrudgingly we accepted the challenge, and the game had begun.

As you might have guessed at this point, my brother and I would spend the rest of that hike, and the others that followed, trying to embody the skills and behaviors that would earn us those cool names we wanted so desperately. We tried to be super quiet, stepping carefully so not to disturb even the smallest twig, or straining and focusing our eyes, in hopes we would spot some wildlife or any other interesting things before anyone else saw them. We tried, mostly in vain, to show off, so that my parents would notice our skills and talents, and in most cases they would pretend not to notice, or offer just slightest encouragement such as, "Wow. You're being so quiet!" Then add, "Do you think you can keep that up for the rest of the hike?"

The exercise worked. From that point on, until we got older and no longer cared, we changed our behavior on the trail and tried to display the best, most resourceful skills we could think of! Even after all that effort we never got new names, but we had a lot fun trying and discussing the options with my dad. In response to our name ideas he would smile and say those dreaded two words parents are known for: "We'll see."

WARNING: *Don't get too tricky with the kids' names and lose the impact of connecting their behavior to the name. Be really explicit, like "Sir Yells A Lot" or "Little Fall Down and Go Boom."*

HINT: *Make sure you give yourself, and any other adults along for the afternoon, really cool names. That way the kids have something to aspire to!*

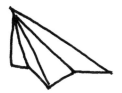

41. FORT CLUB

Keep Kids Busy For:
1–2 hours

You Will Need:
Simple materials from the area

Another great way to get kids to engage with the out-of-doors and have fun all at the same time is building a fort! Take a quick look around you right now. Just scan your immediate area. I'd be willing to bet that if the situation was such that you needed to build a shelter of some kind with just the things around, you could probably do it. Besides, you are the crafty sort.

As kids, my brother and I were always building forts or structures of some kind that we could climb into. Anywhere there was some spare stuff, we'd throw a sheet over it and call it a fort! Whether it was modifying the inside of some bush after a huge snowstorm or stretching blankets over chairs in the living room (see *Occupy The Living Room*), we always had some sort of fort built somewhere to retreat into.

First off, let's get one thing straight. I'm no survivalist. This section on forts is just for fun and by no means am I explaining how to build a shelter in which you could survive the winter or even an over-nighter. Got it? Ok, good. No lawsuits, thank you.

To get started building your own fort, first look around and find a good place to build one. It should offer a little protection or something to build off of, such a fallen tree, a little hill you could tuck up against, some big rocks, or a little wooded area where you could use low-hanging branches. You can probably understand that the right place can take care of a lot of the work of building your fort right off the bat. So, take a little extra time to find a location with the most advantages for your fort-building purposes.

Once you settle on a spot, begin looking for things like big branches, small dead trees, or clumps of dry grass and pine needles. Personally I would also collect heaping piles of pinecones, in preparation for the inevitable pine-cone war that my brother would initiate once we got our forts in working order.

Every once in awhile my dad would build a fort as well. He would get involved for fun, or especially if he thought our interest in building was waning and he needed to step in and stoke our creative juices to keep the ball rolling.

Looking back at it, I'm realizing we usually considered fort building a contest, but no one was doing any judging and there were never any winners. But I do know one thing. We left some pretty cool forts behind on those afternoon adventures. Some of them were even fully outfitted with piles of pinecones ready for battle.

OK, so you picked a spot and loaded up on some basic building materials from the area. Now all you need to do is figure out a way to build up the structure.

First, you need to plot out the size. How wide and how high should it be? In my opinion you should be able to at least lie down in it and also be able to sit up straight on your knees when inside your fort. With all that in mind, let's look at a couple of basic "quick fort" designs.

The Lean-To

The easiest structure to build anywhere is the lean-to. A lean-to could be defined as a temporary structure consisting of a single flat leaning "roof" that extends from a certain height all the way to the ground. The open sides are commonly oriented away from the wind and rain. Lean-tos are often made with found branches and logs and most often used as a camping shelter.

The Lean-To is the most basic "quick fort" to build when you're out having fun in the wilderness. Get a bunch of long branches and lean them against a rock or a tree and you're basically done. Of course, you'll want to keep piling on dry turf and smaller branches to fill up the gaps left by the main branches you started with. Before you know it you've got a great makeshift shelter. Continue adding to it with a floor of collected pine needles, a small wall of collected rocks, or even an additional slanted roof wall.

The Tipi (teepee)

Another easy "quick fort" is the tipi. This free-standing conical structure is made by carefully balancing three or four main posts together and either hoping they won't fall or lashing them together with some kind of rope. I know that the traditional tipi is a tent of poles with a tarp or cloth draped over, but remember, we're out building fun forts and it's a safe bet that no one brought any tent cloth!

Like most "quick forts," once you have the main structural beams in place, you just collect and toss more materials on to seal up the spaces and you're ready to go! These secondary materials should consist of laying down beams across the two main supports and setting more on top of each other to form walls on each side of the structure. Be sure to pick smaller sticks as you get closer to the pointed top of the tipi.

The end of the piled sticks can mesh with the beams of the next wall to help strengthen the tipi.

Once you complete piling up materials to make the walls, then you can toss on more collected materials to fill up spaces and provide more density to the fort.

The Lodge
The final fort I'll talk about here is one that I like to call the lodge. Simply put, a "lodge" is a temporary shelter to be used to hunker down in for a limited amount of time. This "quick fort" relies mainly on some natural topography for a good portion of the structure, more so than the last two. Basically, it's a roof built spanning two large rocks or some natural outcroppings that allow you to get comfortably between and do your hunkering.

If you're lucky enough to find a spot like this, it's not a problem to throw some branches and found beams across the space, and before long you'll be able to get down to the serious job of preparing for any spies and/or saboteurs creeping over from the opposing team.

I'm sure you can easily come up with some other cool designs. If you do, take pictures and email me!

Ultimately, what we parents want is for kids to associate all this family time and the outdoors with fun and fond memories. Building forts and thinking of little games to play is one awesome way to do that.

Good luck and have fun!

WARNING: *There are a couple warnings I'd like to leave you with on this one. First of all, pinecones can hurt. Therefore, aim for the legs. Second, before you go off-trail to build your fort, make sure it's OK to do. Often, the park services would rather you don't stray off the trail because of erosion issues or to protect plant life. It could also be for your protection! Third, only use dry, dead wood and timber. Don't disturb or destroy any living plant life out there just so you can build a dang fort. Fourth, keep an eye peeled for poison ivy or poison oak! And last, if you leave your fort at the end of the day, be sure it's cool. Don't leave a lame fort. Do a good job. If you don't want to leave it and would rather destroy it, then scatter the materials around the area before you leave. Don't leave your fort in a pile. #fortclub*

HINT: *If you're planning on building a fort, bring some gloves. You'll be happy you did! Also bring a Leatherman or a Swiss Army knife. It'll come in handy.*

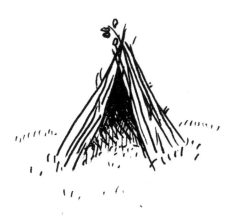

NO LOSERS? NO WINNERS.

This book has been an invitation to look at things a little differently when it comes to your kids and possibly your afternoon drinking. Both require you to be a little more present, perhaps a bit more mindful, and to be willing to see all the things we do and all the stupid little things we say as opportunities to teach valuable and lasting lessons.

WARNING: *All of your creative and smarty-pants parenting techniques and your attempts to make your kids think for themselves could backfire! You might actually be teaching your kids to have an amazing sense of humor and whip out smart problem-solving skills.*

HINT: *Face it. Some of us arrive into parenthood / middle age a little jaded. But luckily for the next generation there are just enough of us out there willing to think outside of the box and try some new tricks, if only to amuse ourselves.*

So, I continue. I feel that tricking them to do the right thing is not only good, but required. I'll keep doing whatever it takes to implant that coveted moral compass in hopes they will stay on the right path even when I'm not around. Cheers. Is there any more wine left?